HEIDI HERMAN
Contribution by Rhonda Thornton

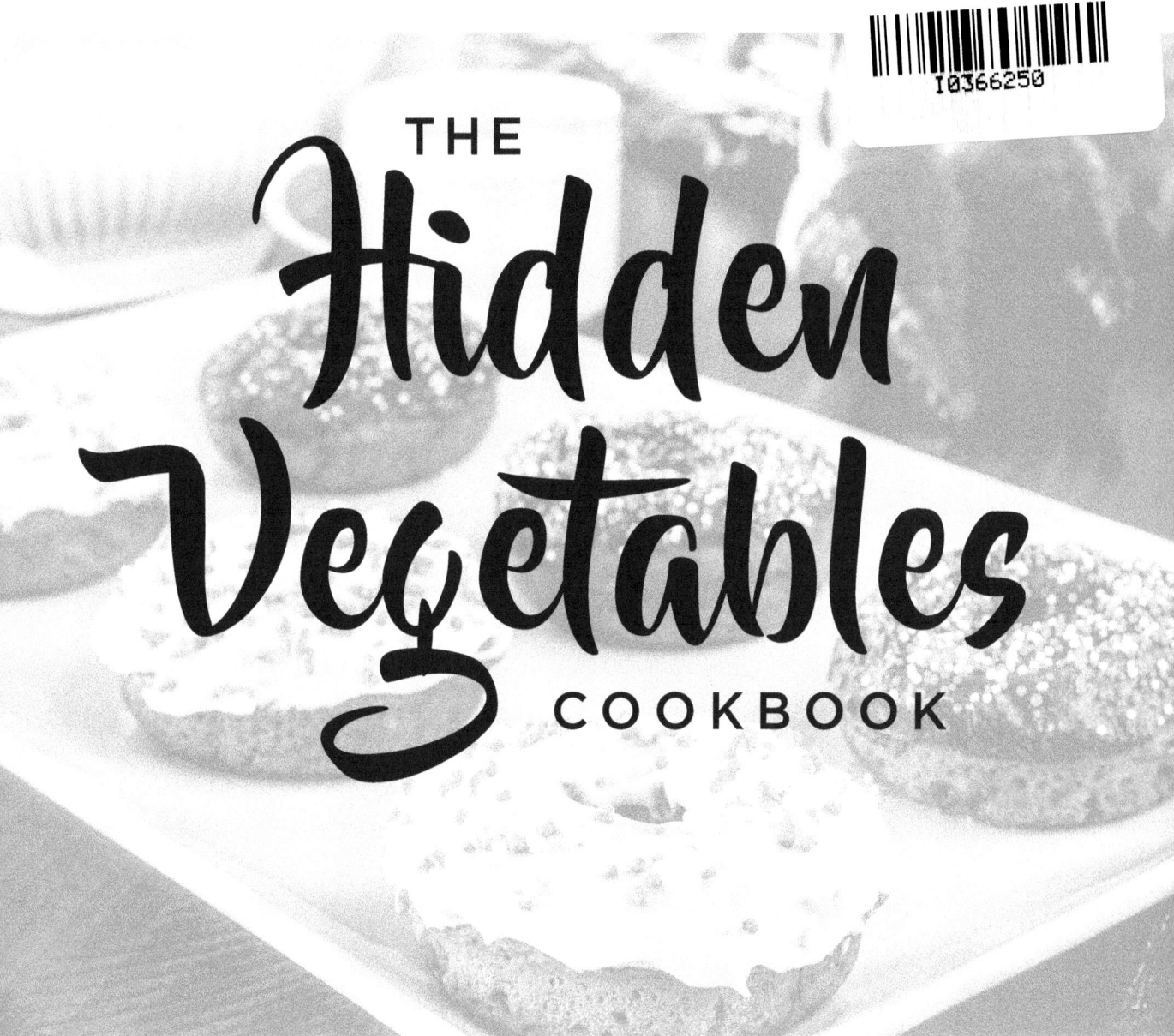

The Hidden Vegetables
COOKBOOK

90 TASTY RECIPES FOR VEGGIE-AVERSE ADULTS

The Hidden Vegetables Cookbook
90 Tasty Recipes for Veggie-Averse Adults
Copyright 2025. All Rights Reserved.
© Heidi Herman

No part of this book may be used or reproduced by any mechanical, photographic, or electronic process, or in the form of a phonograph recording, nor may it be stored in a retrieval system, transmitted, or otherwise copied without the written permission from the author except in the case of brief quotations embodied in critical articles and reviews.

Cook Safely! Make sure you have a clean workspace and keep all of your ingredients properly refrigerated or stored until ready for use. Check the ingredients for each recipe to determine if any ingredient may cause any allergic or other adverse reaction for you or any of your guests.

The author and publisher are not liable for any adverse reactions to food consumed, misinterpreted recipes, or accidents including fires in your kitchen, a cut finger, etc. and they specifically disclaim any liability from the use or application of any of the contents of this book.

The information contained in this cookbook is for informational and entertainment purposes only. This book is not intended to diagnose, treat, cure, or prevent any condition or disease, and nothing contained in this book should be construed as professional or health or medical advice. Readers are solely responsible for their own actions and decisions when preparing and consuming food from this cookbook. Please use your best judgment when using ingredients. If you have questions about a particular condition or possible reactions resulting from the ingredients in a recipe, you should consult with a physician or other qualified health care professional.

Published by:

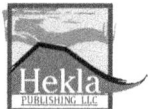

Hekla Publishing LLC,
1603 Capitol Ave Ste 310-A431 Cheyenne, WY 82001
www.heklapublishing.com
Email: info@heklapublishing.com

edited by: Edward Smith and Alice Sage
interior design by: Rebecca Finkel, F + P Graphic Design, FPGD.com
cover design by: Kelly A. Martin KAM.design
© Scott Erb and Donna Dufault photo cover credit

ISBN color hard back: 978-1-947233-11-9
ISBN color paper back: 978-1-947233-12-6
ISBN B&W paper back: 978-1-947233-13-3
ISBN eBook: 978-1-947233-14-0

Library of Congress Control Number: 2025909070

First edition | Printed in USA

Contents

Introduction 1

Why Eat More Vegetables? 6
10 Awesome Reasons to Eat More Veggies 7

Veggie Buying & Storage 8

Using Top-Quality Weapons 19

Varying Methods of Attack 22

Be Versatile and Agile 23

Core Recipes 25

    beets 26
    bell peppers 29
    tomatoes 31
    cauliflower 33
    leeks 34
    onion 35
    kohlrabi 36
    butternut squash 37
    carrots 38
    pumpkin 40
    sweet potato 41
    rutabaga 42
    asparagus 43
    broccoli 44
    Brussels sprouts 45
    celery 46

green peas 47
kale 48
spinach 50
Swiss chard 52
zucchini 53

Uses for Cauliflower and Zucchini Water (Juice) .. 54

Sauces, Spreads & Jellies 55

Appetizers, Soups & Snacks 63

Breads 77

Breakfast 91

Main Dishes 107

Fresh vs Frozen 134

Side Dishes 135

    Fast Veggie-Infused Side Dishes 139

Desserts 149

Index 168

Cooking Measurement Equivalents 171

Emergency Substitutions 172

Spice Substitutions & Alternatives 173

About the Author 174

About the Contributor 174

Introduction

I hate vegetables. There cannot be a truer statement about me. It's their taste, their texture, and with some, even the smell. Yet, as a responsible adult, I know I need to eat my veggies for their significant health benefits.

For years, I heard: "You just need to steam them," "Eat them raw," or "Just start eating them, you'll acquire a taste", and my favorite, "How can you not like them? They're yummy." Nothing I tried made them any more appealing.

Some vegetables make me grimace as I choke them down, others I fight not to spit out, and a few I find impossible to eat because the mere scent makes me gag before I can attempt a taste. At this point, I have accepted that I will never acquire the taste for vegetables. But with the cooking options of a grown-up, I've found a way I can live with that fact, but still benefit from their nutrition.

First things first, though—how did I become veggie-averse?

The Inherited Viking Palate

Growing up, I rarely thought about food or nutrition. But then what kid does except to voice a preference (or aversion)? For me, breakfast was a hurried affair before school, lunch usually from the cafeteria, and dinner a simple meal of soup and sandwich or Hamburger Helper. At least that is what I can recall after forty-plus years.

Sometimes, on a Sunday or holiday, Mom prepared a meal with a main dish, two vegetables, and bread. More often than not, those two vegetables were potatoes and corn, which was pretty typical for the American Midwest where I grew up.

I learned about the food pyramid in school, though I never took it to heart. My mother was from Iceland. She met my father during WWII when he was stationed there, and after they married, she immigrated to the United States. She would often say that green vegetables were rabbit food —not something they ate in Iceland. Instead, their nutrition came from fish, seafood, and dairy. That, and the cod liver oil they were dosed with every morning at school!

I patterned my eating habits after Mom's. My palate was influenced by what she liked and didn't like. She rarely served vegetables when I was young, so I wasn't one of those kids who were forced to eat vegetables. As a result, I never developed a taste for them. Mom ate an occasional green salad but was never a fan of vegetables either. At one physical, she said the doctor wanted her to add more greens to her diet. So, she went straight to the grocery store and bought a big bag of M&M's to sort out all the green ones. Doctor's orders, she laughed.

But it wasn't just her food habits that influenced me. I also inherited her lifelong deep love of both reading and writing. At the age of 88, she wrote and self-published a memoir, *Growing Up Viking*, about her Icelandic childhood.

Following her example, I was inspired to create several books inspired by my Icelandic heritage while she continued to write as well. We established a small publishing company and traveled together promoting our books and Icelandic culture. At that point, with Mom over ninety years old, wherever we went, a common theme in the questions directed at her was: "Where do you get your energy?" "Wow—you're so active and how old?" and "How do you maintain such vitality?"

She often brushed off such questions but confided to me that she didn't want to disclose her secret because she didn't want to make people feel bad. She truly believed her vitality was due to her Scandinavian heritage—her Viking Blood, as she called it. She insisted it was the reason she could remain active, energetic, and maintain a healthy weight.

These were all attributes that I wanted to emulate—but what if it wasn't all genetic?

Embrace the Distaste

As an adult, I endured ribbing from my colleagues at professional lunches when I'd pass on the salad or leave my plate virtually licked-clean on one side and the other side, where the vegetables sat, completely untouched.

After forty, I began to realize the importance of nutrition, which I was probably lacking. I wasn't living in Iceland as my mother had in her early years; I didn't have a steady diet of fresh fish or raw dairy. Honestly, I'd become a carboholic—and it was starting to catch up with me. Twenty years prior, I underwent back surgery and became accustomed to at least a minimal amount of related pain or stiffness. But, after my midlife milestone, my energy level diminished, I suffered from headaches, foggy brain, and overall aches and pains increased.

My doctor suggested it was chronic inflammation or just natural aging. He recommended supplements, and I had to admit it was time to embrace the importance of vitamins and minerals for my health. While researching my 2020 book, *On With the Butter! Spread More Living onto Everyday Life*[1], I started to understand the broader impact food has on overall health. The more studies I read, the more I wanted to learn. This period of food education changed the way I approached ingredients in my kitchen. The following is an excerpt from a chapter in that book entitled "Taste Life:"

> "We all know that food provides us with nutrition that fuels our bodies and keeps us healthy. We also know it's important to get the recommended amounts of nutrients and limit the indulgences that aren't good for us so that we can maintain a healthy heart, a strong immune system, and good overall health. But recent studies indicate that what we eat can also affect our moods and mental health.

---

[1] Heidi Herman, *On With the Butter! Spread More Living onto Everyday Life*, Hekla Publishing 2020, p. 90-91

In 2015, a study published in Harvard Health, a publication of Harvard Medical School, showed that while the digestive system's primary function is to process food, the gastrointestinal tract produces almost all the serotonin in our body. Serotonin has a critical function in regulating sleep and controlling appetite, but it also plays a role in maintaining healthy moods and inhibiting pain.

Staying physically healthy, sleeping well, and keeping balanced moods are all good reasons to strive for a healthy diet. But balanced nutrition—antioxidants and B vitamins are especially important—might also help to preserve brain function. Studies from Harvard's Brigham and Women's Hospital, Johns Hopkins University, and UCLA have shown that certain "brain foods" may slow the loss of cognitive function and memory and might even improve memory. Brain foods include green vegetables, fatty fish, berries, and walnuts.

But as we age, our sensitivity for both taste and smell diminishes, and our favorite foods can become less appealing. That can lead to eating less and not getting the nutrition we need, so it's important to find the balance between nutritional benefit and enjoyment."

I knew nutrition was important, but I never realized just how important. General well-being, less pain, fewer aches and pains, better sleep, sharper mental function, the list goes on and on. Well, who wouldn't want all these things and more? It became more than just about anti-inflammation. That realization brought a focus on the long-term quality of life.

Since both my parents lived into their early 90's, I knew there was a long life ahead of me and if I wanted to be able to enjoy it fully, I must make some changes. I needed balanced nutrition, and that included more vegetables, particularly the ones I disliked the most. Spinach, Kale, Beets, Broccoli—all those crucial veggies I'd literally turned up my nose at—were the foundation of my healthy future.

To achieve this healthy future, I needed to incorporate more fresh, nutritionally dense foods into my diet. But my goal wasn't to learn how to like vegetables, it was simply to eat more of them. I needed to embrace the distaste and own it.

The Kitchen Viking

It was an epiphany, yet simple. I didn't have to like vegetables. I only had to accept being veggie-averse and align that with my desire to eat more nutritious food. I am a self-taught cook and enjoyed being in the kitchen, so that was a start. I excelled at creating tasty cookies and baked goods—I just needed to expand my horizons a bit. I decided to reach back into my ancestry for inspiration. I would begin exploration, apply a little creative craftsmanship, and ultimately conquer vegetables. I was a kitchen Viking embarking on a veggie voyage.

To do that, I decided to employ Viking Law #1:

Be Brave and Aggressive

Be direct

Grab all opportunities

Use varying methods of attack

Be versatile and agile

Attack one target at a time

Don't plan everything in detail

Use top quality weapons

I could directly apply this approach to the preparation and incorporation of vegetables into my diet. And thus began my journey. I started working on adapting some of my favorite dishes as well as creating new ones with a twist towards more nutrition.

I collected hundreds of cookbooks, scouring recipes for ideas, and went down rabbit holes of research, and experimenting with ways to prepare vegetables that were tolerable to my palate. In the process, I developed some recipes that are downright tasty. I even discovered that a few of the veggies are not nearly as bad as I thought they were, and that some have flavors that disappear entirely when mixed with other ingredients.

Naturally, it wasn't all successful. The results of some experiments were truly awful. My dear mother was such a sport in taste-testing. The kale cinnamon rolls weren't so bad, she said, if you dipped them in coffee. (That was one recipe that didn't make the cut for this cookbook!) My husband was more honest. He decreed that my first three attempts with Brussels sprouts were "a terrible thing to do to bacon."

However, I persevered and eventually found ways to incorporate fresh, healthy vegetables into the food I loved without compromising the flavor or texture. I discovered that Brussels sprouts exude a nutty flavor and remain crunchy, so pairing them with walnuts and honey in rice was perfect. The sweet, nutty crunch just added more flavor and texture, and the Brussels sprouts blended in the background. Cauliflower rice—popular in recent years—seemed like a good go-to, but I could never disguise the flavor enough until I started adding ginger. A small but magical adjustment.

Vegetable Sneakery

It has taken years to incorporate more vegetables into my diet. Guess what? I still hate some of them—in their raw, natural form anyway. In the end, my assessment was that: there are a few veggies I have no problem enjoying, others need some flavor enhancements, but the bulk needed to be deeply hidden. That's where vegetable sneakery comes in.

As I shared my findings with friends and associates, I finally understood I wasn't alone in my adulthood vegetable-averseness. But it wasn't until I read a 2022 *New York Post* article[2] about how people thought a healthy lifestyle would make them miserable that I truly realized how many people dislike vegetables. One phrase from the article stuck with me—that "being healthy … meant eating food that's bad on the taste buds but good for their bodies." That was a lightbulb moment. I knew then that I had to assemble these recipes into book form to help people like me eat their vegetables while still loving their food.

After fifteen years of experimenting, I still don't love my vegetables, but you would never know that when I'm in the grocery check-out lane, pushing a cart piled high with fresh produce. Even better, I eat it all too! If you ever dine at my home, you may not be able to identify which dish is veggie-infused, and that's worth all the time I spent wrangling vegetables.

So, if you are like me—veggie-averse but health-focused—here are a few pointers. The first is to be open to taste-testing. If the vegetable in question is something you like, great. If not, take the time to assess whether your issue is with the smell, flavor (or lack thereof), or texture. Afterward, you can decide on how to (or if indeed you wish to) sneak that particular one into your diet. Be open to experimenting with different spices and flavors. It's a journey, so make it fun!

My hope is that you will enjoy this cookbook and the ideas it offers for adding a little nutritional kick to dishes you and your whole family can love—even if they never love the vegetables.

—Heidi Herman

---

a note on Portions, Servings, and Yields

A **serving size** is a defined, measured quantity of food used for nutritional information, like on a food label. This measurement is established by the U.S. Food and Drug Administration (FDA) based on the actual amounts of food and beverages that people do consume, rather than what they should consume.

In cookbooks, it's typical for recipes to specify the **number of portions** or servings, indicating how much food a particular recipe is designed to serve. Like the FDA guidelines, these portion sizes can often be misleading, leaving us confused about what an appropriate amount to eat really is. Why is that? Firstly, personal factors play a significant role in determining how much food we should eat. Elements such as metabolism, age, weight, height, activity level, and even dietary restrictions all influence what is deemed a suitable portion. Secondly, the overall meal plan can impact individual portion sizes. For instance, a serving of casserole might be larger per person if it is served without accompanying side dishes.

Given these complexities, I have intentionally chosen not to specify exact portions for most recipes in this cookbook. However, where relevant, I have noted the **Yield,** which refers to the quantity that a recipe produces, such as one medium kohlrabi yielding about two cups of diced kohlrabi.

---

[2] https://nypost.com/2022/07/14/most-people-think-a-healthy-lifestyle-will-make-them-miserable/

Why Eat More Vegetables?

Rhonda Thornton National Board Certified Health and Wellness Coach, Senior Fitness Specialist, Certified Personal Trainer, Corrective Exercise Specialist, Master Certified Life Coach, and Diabetes Paraprofessional Career Path Educator.

Let's be honest—vegetables don't always get a fair shot. As a National Board Certified Health and Wellness Coach, I meet a lot of adults who say they just don't like veggies. And hey, I get it. Some of us grew up thinking of vegetables as boiled, bland, or buried under a pile of cheese. But this cookbook? It's changing the game.

I love that this book takes the pressure off and makes vegetables fun again. Because when you sneak them into meals in creative ways, you're not just feeding your body—you're giving it superpowers. Think of veggies as the unsung heroes of your plate: full of vitamins, minerals, antioxidants, and fiber that help your body thrive.

The USDA says adults should aim for 2 to 3 cups of vegetables a day. But if we're aiming for awesome (not just average), then 3 to 5 cups—or more—is where the magic happens. And guess what? That's totally doable when you add veggies to smoothies, wraps, stir-fries, eggs, soups, or even sauces. Little by little, they add up—and so do the benefits.

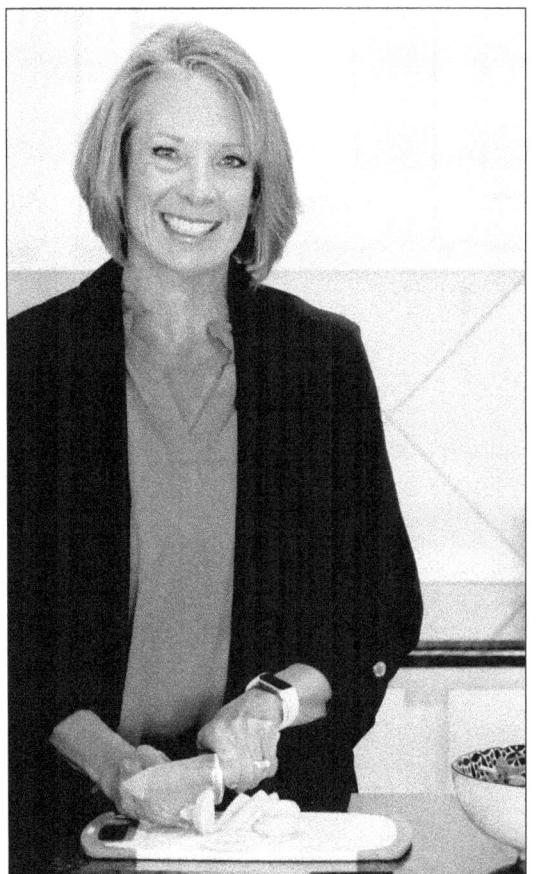

Not a veggie lover yet? No problem. Start small. It's not about perfection—it's about progress. Your body will thank you, your energy will skyrocket, and you just might start craving kale (yes, really).

Why Vegetables Matter
(Even If You Don't Like Them)

Vegetables aren't just a healthy side dish, they're foundational to a vibrant, energized, and disease-resistant life. Packed with powerful plant compounds, fiber, and nutrients, vegetables nourish your body from the inside out. They help your organs function, your digestion work smoothly, and your cells repair and defend themselves daily.

What many people don't realize is that vegetables offer different types of support depending on their color, texture, and flavor profile. Green leafy vegetables are rich in magnesium and calcium, which support muscle and bone health. Orange vegetables like sweet potatoes and squash contain beta-carotene, a precursor to vitamin A, which boosts vision and immunity. Red and purple vegetables like tomatoes and red cabbage offer heart-healthy antioxidants that fight oxidative stress.

Beyond physical health, vegetables impact how we feel. People who eat more vegetables tend to report better moods, more stable energy, and less anxiety. That's partly because fiber feeds your gut microbiome—which plays a huge role in mental health—and partly because your blood sugar stays more balanced. Stable blood sugar means fewer cravings, less brain fog, and more consistent energy throughout the day.

So if you're someone who has struggled to get enough vegetables in, you're not alone. But small, consistent changes—like sneaking spinach into a smoothie—can completely shift how your body feels and functions. It's not about perfection. It's about building a life that supports your goals, one veggie at a time.

As a National Board Certified Health and Wellness Coach who specializes in nutrition for adults, I'm thrilled to see a cookbook created specifically for adults who don't like vegetables. In my coaching practice, I've worked with many clients who tell me they just can't get into vegetables—but I know how powerful these foods can be for energy, vitality, and overall health.

10 Awesome Reasons to Eat More Veggies

They're like a **multivitamin from nature**—boosting your immune system and energy levels.

Your gut **loves** them. Fiber feeds your good bacteria, keeping digestion smooth and happy.

They **help fight inflammation,** which is linked to everything from joint pain to brain fog.

They **keep things moving** (you know what I mean)—hello, better digestion!

They **help stabilize blood sugar** and curb those wild snack attacks.

They're **heart heroes**—lowering cholesterol and blood pressure naturally.

They **protect your eyes** with nutrients like beta-carotene and lutein.

They **give you glowing skin** from the inside out (vitamins A and C, baby!).

They **help you feel full, satisfied, and fueled**—not sluggish.

They **help lower the risk of big scary stuff like heart disease, diabetes, and cancer.**

Veggie Buying & Storing

A significant part of my vegetable journey involved learning how to select, store, and handle fresh produce. I often ventured online after coming across a previously unknown vegetable to answer the question:

"What in the world do I do with this?"

I thought it might be helpful to include this section to share some of the insights and tidbits of information I've collected over the years. Some wisdom comes from the heartfelt advice of wise women and seasoned gardeners, while others are gems from online research, helpful household tips publications, and my beloved cookbook collection.

If you are like me and not so knowledgeable about vegetables, this section may guide you in selecting vegetables at the market or produce stand, storing them until you have time to make your core recipes, and preserving them for longer-term storage. To help with choosing which ones to try, I've included notes on what they taste like, how their texture feels, and what nutritional benefit each one may provide. Finally, I've listed the spices and flavors that each veggie either blends well with or, as I've found, does the best job of disguising its particular flavor.

I am not a produce expert or formally educated in this area, and some of the information may be outdated or incorrect. I encourage you to verify and update it as needed. After all, the best cookbooks are those that feature dog-ears, underlines, or handwritten notes in the margins!

Asparagus

Selecting Asparagus should have a deep or vibrant green color and may have a slight purplish tinge on the tips. Spears should be straight and firm. They should not be limp, bendable or rubbery, or wilted-looking. They also should not have dry, cracked ends. The tips should be closed.

Source For asparagus in season, a farmers' market will usually have fresher produce that is typically sweeter, juicier, and more tender than at the grocery store. Peak season is April through June.

Short-Term Storage When you bring it home, rinse and shake off excess water. If you have room in the refrigerator, asparagus will stay freshest when stored standing upright in water. Another alternative is to wrap it in a damp paper towel, place it in a plastic bag, and lay it flat in the refrigerator.

Will keep short-term for up to three days.

Long-Term Storage Asparagus can be frozen but is often watery and limp when thawed. Trimming, cleaning, and puréeing before freezing may give the best results when thawed.

Flavor The common green asparagus is earthy with a grassy or leaf-like flavor. Many people think it tastes similar to green peas, but it has a distinctly different texture. The thinner stalks are more tender, while thicker, larger stalks are tougher with a "woody" Flavor and can often taste bitter. White asparagus is sweeter and has a milder flavor.

Texture Raw asparagus is firm and should be crispy. Steamed asparagus spears are smooth and will have a slight crispness. Overcooked asparagus will be mushy and soft.

Asparagus (continued)

Spices and Herbs that Blend Well or Disguise

Garlic Powder	Lemon Peel
Chili Flakes	Black Pepper
Paprika	Rosemary
Thyme	Dill

Nutritional Benefits Good source of fiber; rich in vitamins A, C, E, & K; and contains prebiotics, folate, potassium, magnesium, and chromium.

Beets

Selecting Beets should be maroon-colored with green leaves, but it's okay if the greens have been cut off. The bulbs should still have a thin, pointed root attached, but avoid ones with hairy roots because they're likely older and will have a woodier flavor. Choose ones that are 2" to 3" in diameter with smooth, unblemished skin. The smaller ones will be more difficult to peel, and the larger ones are tougher with a woodier flavor. They should be firm and not feel mushy.

Source Available year-round at the grocery store, beets are usually seen at farmers' markets or local produce stands during peak season, that is, late summer to late fall.

Short-Term Storage When you bring them home, trim the greens. Wash the beets, wrap them in paper towels, and store them in a plastic bag in the refrigerator. Trimmed greens will keep 1–2 days in the refrigerator.

Whole beets will keep for 3–4 weeks.

Long-Term Storage For trimmed greens, wash and rinse. Dice and package in a freezer-safe bag in the freezer. Will keep for 6 to 12 months.

For the beets, roast, peel, and slice, then lay flat in a single layer in freezer-safe or vacuum-sealed bags. Will keep frozen for 6 to 12 months. Take them out to purée or juice.

Flavor Beets have an earthy flavor, and for some, they taste like "dirt." They can be slightly sweet and sometimes have a bitter flavor.

Texture Beets are crunchy when raw and have a smooth, buttery texture when cooked. Greens are crisp when raw and smooth when puréed.

Spices and Herbs that Blend Well or Disguise

Red Wine vinegar/Balsamic vinegar	
Salt	Rosemary
Thyme	Citrus juice

Nutritional Benefits Good source of antioxidants and fiber and contains folate, vitamin C, manganese, and iron.

Bell Peppers

Selecting Peppers should be firm and well-shaped and have vibrant colors with a glossy look. They should not have dark spots, holes, wrinkled skin, or a wilted stem. Young peppers will be green and have the strongest flavors. Green peppers will turn yellow, orange, or red as they mature, and they will get sweeter. Red peppers have the highest nutrients.

Source Readily available at farmers' markets in season, typically June–September. Often, bell peppers will be less expensive at a grocery store, and organic options are usually comparable to farmers' markets.

Short-Term Storage Place unwashed whole peppers in a breathable bag like mesh, cotton, or muslin, and store them in the crisper drawer of the refrigerator but not in the same drawer as fruits.

Uncut peppers will keep for 1–2 weeks in the refrigerator.

Long-Term Storage Wash, remove stems and seeds, and dice. Place in vacuum-sealed bags and freeze; will keep for up to 12 months.

Flavor Red peppers will have the sweetest flavor, but all varieties may taste bitter. Bell peppers are typically juicy, especially when raw.

Bell Peppers (continued)

Texture Firm, crispy texture when raw; softer when cooked but will still have some bite. Often undetectable when diced.

Spices and Herbs that Blend Well or Disguise

- Salt
- Sugar
- Honey
- Lemon juice
- Soy sauce

Nutritional Benefits Good source of vitamins A & C, fiber, and antioxidants.

Broccoli

Selecting Broccoli comes in bunches that should have firm, short stalks and dark green to bluish-green heads with firm, compact florets. Avoid any with wilted stems, yellow or orange spots, or loose florets.

Source Typically available year-round at grocery stores and will likely be less expensive there than at farmers' markets or produce stands. Peak harvest season will vary by region and depends on planting time, but can be October through April.

Short-Term Storage Place unwashed whole broccoli in a plastic bag with holes for airflow, close loosely, and store in the crisper drawer of the refrigerator—but not in the same drawer as fruit—for 5 to 7 days.

Long-Term Storage Wash and pat dry. Dice stalks, heads, and florets. Place in vacuum-sealed bags and freeze for up to 12 months.

Flavor Broccoli has an earthy or grassy flavor and is often bitter. The stalk of the broccoli usually has a milder flavor than the florets. Both parts will usually have a milder flavor but a stronger smell when cooked. Broccoli is one of the cruciferous vegetables that has sulfur-containing compounds that get stronger when the vegetable is chopped, cooked, or chewed, all of which release the compound, increasing the smell and associated flavor, which can be unpleasant.

Texture The texture of the florets can be crumbly; stalks are crisp and crunchy unless overcooked, in which case they can be mushy.

Spices and Herbs that Blend Well or Disguise

- Garlic
- Red pepper flakes
- Honey
- Maple syrup
- Rosemary

Nutritional Benefits Broccoli contains antioxidants; vitamins A, C, & K; calcium; and potassium and is high in fiber.

Brussels sprouts

Selecting Brussels sprouts should be firm, and the leaves closed. Avoid ones with brown spots and loose or wilted leaves. Smaller, yellow ones will have a milder flavor.

Source Farmers' markets will usually have fresher Brussels sprouts than grocery stores. This is best because fresher Sprouts are sweeter, and they get bitter the longer they stay on the shelves. You're also more likely to find some with stems attached, which will make them last much longer. However, they're typically available year-round in grocery stores.

Short-Term Storage If there are stems, trim the sprouts slightly then place them upright in water and refrigerate. Without stems, bag and remove any wilted or brown leaves. Place unwashed and whole in an air-tight food storage container or a sealed plastic bag and store in the crisper drawer of the refrigerator, but not in the same drawer as fruit, for 5 to 7 days.

Long-Term Storage Wash, blanch, and freeze whole in vacuum-sealed bags or wash, dice completely, and then place in vacuum-sealed bags and freeze for up to 12 months.

Flavor Earthy, nutty, bitter flavor similar to cabbage. Smaller, yellow ones will have a milder flavor. Brussels sprouts is one of the cruciferous vegetables that have sulfur-containing compounds that get stronger upon chopping, cooking, or chewing, all of which release the compound. This increases the smell and associated flavor, which can be unpleasant.

Texture Crisp and crunchy, even when cooked.

Spices and Herbs that Blend Well or Disguise

Honey	Brown Sugar
Balsamic Vinegar	Lemon Juice
Red Pepper Flakes	

Nutritional Benefits High in fiber, vitamins K & C, and rich in antioxidants.

Butternut Squash

Selecting It should feel heavy and dense. The skin should be matte dark beige, not glossy, and have a firm, dry stem. Squash should be firm without soft spots, cuts, or discoloration.

Source Readily available at many farmers' markets and produce stands; peak harvest season is August to November. Typically available year-round in grocery stores.

Short-Term Storage Store uncut squash in a cool, dark, dry spot outside the fridge like a cupboard or root cellar, ideally at 50 to 60 degrees fahrenheit for up to 3 months, but do not store alongside fruits.

Long-Term Storage Cut, roast, and chop or purée, place in vacuum-sealed bags, and freeze for 8 to 12 months.

Flavor Flavor is mild, and often bitter if cut too close to the rind. It has a buttery, nutty, and slightly sweet flavor, similar to sweet potato or pumpkin.

Texture Raw squash is firm and crunchy. When cooked, it is smooth and starchy, but a bit thicker than a baked potato.

Spices and Herbs that Blend Well or Disguise

Sweet: Cinnamon, Nutmeg

Savory: Cumin, Coriander, Cayenne Pepper

Nutritional Benefits Rich in antioxidants, vitamins A & C, fiber, and potassium.

Carrots

Selecting Should be firm, without any mushy sections. They should be bright orange and have smooth skin without excessive cracks (some are fine). Avoid ones with root hair or brown spots. *Tip:* buying larger packages labeled for juicing can be less expensive. Those packages tend to have larger, less uniform carrots with a few cracks or imperfections, so they're rejected for commercial packaging but are still fine.

Source A basic staple like carrots will often be less expensive at the grocery store and much the same quality, especially if you choose organic. But farmers' markets are always a great option for carrots.

Short-Term Storage Remove any attached greens. Place unwashed, unpeeled carrots in an airtight or sealed plastic bag in the crisper drawer of the refrigerator separate from fruits to keep up to 2 months.

Long-Term Storage Peel, clean before chopping, and blanch or dice in a food processor to freeze. Lay flat in freezer-safe or vacuum-sealed bags. Will keep frozen for 9 to 12 months.

Flavor Raw carrots have an earthy taste that is sweet and more, becoming even more mild when cooked.

Texture Raw carrots are firm and crunchy but become soft when baked or steamed.

Spices and Herbs that Blend Well or Disguise

Many spices will cut the bitterness or overwhelm the mild flavor of carrots.

Cinnamon or nutmeg	Honey
Garlic	Coriander

Nutritional Benefits Carrots provide a good source of vitamins A & C, potassium, and fiber.

Cauliflower

Selecting A head of cauliflower should be uniform in color, overall creamy-white without brown spots. They should feel firm, with tightly packed heads and no soft spots. If there are leaves, they should not be brown or wilting.

Source A basic staple like cauliflower will often be less expensive at the grocery store and much the same quality, especially if you choose organic. A farmers' market or produce stand is always a great option for cauliflower.

Short-Term Storage Store whole, unwashed heads of cauliflower in a loosely closed or perforated plastic bag in the crisper drawer of the refrigerator, placed stem side up, for 3 to 4 weeks.

Long-Term Storage Clean and rice to prepare before freezing. Lay flat in freezer-safe or vacuum-sealed bags for 9 to 12 months.

Flavor In general, cauliflower has a mild flavor, which some describe as slightly nutty or peppery. Cauliflower is one of the cruciferous vegetables that has sulfur-containing compounds that get stronger when chopped, cooked, or chewed, all of which release the compound. This increases the smell and associated flavor, which can be unpleasant.

Texture Raw cauliflower is crisp and crunchy, but softens as it cooks. Riced cauliflower may have a pebbly consistency, or be nearly undistinguishable when cooked to softness.

Spices and Herbs that Blend Well or Disguise

Garlic	Paprika
Chili Powder	Ginger
Onion Powder	

Nutritional Benefits Cauliflower contains vitamins C & K, folate, fiber, and antioxidants.

Celery

Selecting Celery is often sold prepackaged in plastic, which should feel heavy. The stalks should be firm, packed together, and pale green. Avoid any celery that looks wilted, has yellow or brown patches, or feels rubbery.

Source A basic staple like celery will often be less expensive at the grocery store and much the same quality, especially if you choose organic. Farmers' markets and produce stands are excellent sources of celery.

Short-Term Storage Prepackaged celery can be stored in its original packaging for 1 to 2 weeks in the refrigerator crisper drawer. To keep it fresh for as long as a month, remove the celery from the plastic bag, wrap it loosely in a damp paper towel, and then securely in aluminum foil before placing it in the crisper drawer.

Long-Term Storage Wash, trim, and cut into 2-inch pieces. Store in freezer-safe or vacuum-sealed bags. Freeze for up to 12 months.

Flavor Celery has a grassy or mildly earthy flavor and is slightly bitter. The darker the shade of green is, the stronger its flavor will be.

Texture Raw celery is crisp and crunchy with a high water content, while cooked celery softens and may be nearly undistinguishable in soups or stews.

Spices and Herbs that Blend Well or Disguise

Paprika	Parsley
Basil	Rosemary

Nutritional Benefits Celery is a good source of fiber; vitamins A, C, & K; potassium; and folate and is high in antioxidants.

Green Peas

Selecting Green peas are commonly called Sugar Snap Peas and are sold fresh in the pod. Shelled peas are typically sold frozen or canned. Choose ones where the pod looks green, plump, and curvy. The pods should show the contours of the peas and feel full. Avoid dry pods or those with brown or yellow coloring.

Source Fresh peas are typically available from grocery stores. Farmers' markets and produce stands are excellent sources of fresher green peas.

Short-Term Storage Keep peas in the pod and store refrigerated for 2 to 3 days.

Long-Term Storage Shell the peas, rinse under cold water, and pat dry. Store in freezer-safe or vacuum-sealed bags. Freeze for up to 12 months.

Flavor Peas have a light grassy, sweet flavor. To some, the flavor is similar to asparagus but with a distinct texture.

Texture Peas are round and smooth, with a slight bite and soft center. Overcooked peas will be mushy.

Spices and Herbs that Blend Well or Disguise

Mint	Thyme
Rosemary	Dill
Curry	

Nutritional Benefits Peas are a good source of vitamins C & K, protein, fiber, and folate.

Kale

Selecting Kale is typically sold prepackaged or in bunches. Choose kale with bright, deeply colored leaves that are firm and plump. Avoid any that look wilted, discolored, or slimy.

Source Available year-round in the grocery store, Kale is are usually available at farmers' markets or local produce stands during peak season, late summer to late fall.

Short-Term Storage Kale can be stored unwashed, loosely wrapped in a plastic bag in the crisper drawer, or wrapped in a damp paper towel and put in a sealed container in the refrigerator to stay fresh for 5 to 7 days.

Long-Term Storage Wash, blanch, and freeze whole in vacuum-sealed bags or wash, dice completely, or purée then place in vacuum-sealed bags and freeze for up to 12 months.

Flavor Raw kale is often described as earthy, slightly bitter, and sometimes peppery. The flavor is milder if it's picked younger; kale that is older when picked is stronger. Kale is one of the cruciferous vegetables that have sulfur-containing compounds that get stronger when chopped, cooked, or chewed, all of which release the compound, increasing the smell and associated flavor that can be unpleasant. Cooked kale tends to have a milder flavor.

Texture Raw kale is often tough, chewy, and fibrous, but when cooked it becomes tender. Overcooked kale can be soggy or slimy, but puréed is typically smooth.

Spices and Herbs that Blend Well or Disguise and Offset Bitterness

Garlic	Red chili flakes
Paprika	Lemon or Lime juice

Nutritional Benefits Kale has vitamins A, C, & K and is rich in potassium, omega-3 fatty acids, and fiber.

Kohlrabi

Selecting Kohlrabi should be firm and free of discoloration, cracks, or blemishes, and may be green or purple. If there are leaves attached, they should not be wilted. Small sizes, usually less than 3 inches in diameter, are more tender.

Source Kohlrabi is often available in larger grocery stores year-round and at farmers' markets or local produce stands during peak season, fall to early winter, depending on location.

Short-Term Storage Remove leaves from the bulb and wash to remove any dirt or debris. Wrap loosely in a damp paper towel, then in a container with a sealed lid. Place in the crisper drawer for up to 2 or 3 weeks. Use the kohlrabi before it becomes soft.

Long-Term Storage Freezing will allow kohlrabi to stay fresh for up to a year and will make it more tender after thawing. Remove leaves, wash, then blanch for 1 to 2 minutes. Immerse in an ice water bath, pat dry, then seal in airtight freezer bags.

Flavor Raw kohlrabi has a mild but sweet and peppery flavor that is more subtle when cooked.

Texture Raw kohlrabi is crisp, crunchy, and juicy but the texture is slightly rubbery. Cooked kohlrabi is softer.

Spices and Herbs that Blend Well or Disguise and Offset Bitterness

Chili Powder	Paprika
Cumin	

Nutritional Benefits Kohlrabi is rich in potassium, vitamin C, fiber, and beta-carotene.

Leeks

Selecting Leeks should have straight, bright green tops with a white base. They should not be shriveled, brown, or wilted at the top, and the bottom should not be yellow.

Source Leeks are typically available in grocery stores year-round and at farmers' markets or local produce stands during peak season in the fall.

Short-Term Storage Leeks can be stored unwashed in a plastic bag in the crisper drawer of the refrigerator for up to a week.

Long-Term Storage Trim all the tough, dark green leaves and white roots. Keep only the white and light-green parts and discard the rest. Wash thoroughly several times under cold running water. Dry. Dice and freeze in airtight freezer bags.

Flavor Leeks are similar in taste to onions but much milder, and slightly sweet. To some, there may be a mild garlic flavor.

Texture Raw leeks are crunchy and smooth, cooked they become tender and soft.

Spices and Herbs that Blend Well or Disguise

Caraway seeds	Paprika
Coriander	Basil
Garlic	

Nutritional Benefits Leeks are high in vitamins A, C, & K and are a good source of beta-carotene, iron, and antioxidants.

Onion

Selecting Onion may be red, white, or yellow but should generally be uniform in color. It should feel firm without soft spots or discoloration.

Source A basic staple like onion will often be less expensive at the grocery store and much the same quality, especially if you choose organic. Farmers' markets and produce stands may have fresher selections available in season.

Short-Term Storage Once peeled and cut, store onions in a sealed container in the refrigerator for 1 to 2 weeks.

Long-Term Storage Store onions in a cool, dark, and dry place like a pantry or cellar. Allow ventilation using a wire basket or mesh bag to keep them fresh for up to 6–8 months. Leave the skin on, do not refrigerate, and do not store with potatoes. May be cleaned, diced, and frozen in airtight packaging for up to a year.

Flavor Onions can be pungent, with a flavor that is sharp, spicy, tangy, or sweet depending on the variety.

Texture Raw onions have a dry, thin, and papery exterior. Inner layers are thicker, smooth, and maybe crunchy or soft and juicy depending on the variety. Cooked onions will become soft and may be undiscernible in cooked dishes when diced.

Spices and Herbs that Blend Well or Disguise

Ginger	Garlic
Sugar or honey	

Nutritional Benefits Onions are rich in vitamin C, potassium, and folate.

Pumpkin

Selecting Pumpkins should have a vibrant, bright orange color. The rind should be firm and hard, without soft spots, cuts, or blemishes. It should have a well-attached dry, brown stem.

Source Often plentiful and available at grocery stores year-round and at farmers' markets or produce stands in the fall, from September through November.

Short-Term Storage Pumpkins should be stored whole, fresh, and uncut in a cool, dry, well-ventilated place like a pantry, cellar, or garage. It should be stored away from apples, pears, or other ripening fruits to stay fresh for several months.

Long-Term Storage When properly cleaned and processed, pumpkin can be frozen to stay fresh for up to a year.

Flavor Fresh pumpkin has a mild flavor, often described as earthy, slightly sweet, or nutty.

Texture The outside of a pumpkin is firm and smooth, but the inside soft flesh, which is more commonly eaten, is typically smooth when baked or puréed.

Spices and Herbs that Blend Well

Cinnamon	Nutmeg
Ginger	Cloves

Nutritional Benefits Pumpkins are rich in vitamins A & K, beta-carotene, and fiber.

Rutabaga

Selecting Rutabaga should be firm to the touch, round or oval in shape, with smooth unblemished skin. Avoid any with soft spots or cracks. Large ones will be more bitter, so it's best to choose the ones about 3-inches to 5-inches in diameter.

Source Often plentiful and available at grocery stores year-round and at farmers' markets or produce stands often in the fall.

Short-Term Storage Wipe away any excess dirt or debris. Wrap whole, unwashed rutabagas in a moist paper towel then place in a perforated plastic bag or a vegetable storage bag in the crisper drawer of the refrigerator to store for up to a month.

Stored in a cool, dry, well-ventilated area like a root cellar or basement, they can stay fresh for several months. Do not allow them to touch and check them every few weeks to ensure they haven't started to spoil.

Long-Term Storage *To freeze:* Peel, cut into cubes, blanch in boiling water for 3 minutes, and then cool in ice water. Dry. Seal in airtight freezer bags, but do not overfill. Frozen rutabaga will keep for 6 months to a year.

Flavor The flavor is mild. Raw, a rutabaga is similar to a turnip but slightly sweeter and not as bitter. Cooked, a rutabaga is sweeter and similar to a baked potato.

Texture Raw rutabaga is crisp and crunchy, but once cooked it is soft and smooth.

Spices that Blend Well

Paprika	Cumin
Garlic	Fennel Seeds

Nutritional Benefits Rutabaga is an excellent source of vitamins C & E, potassium, and magnesium.

Spinach

Selecting Spinach should have vibrant green leaves without brown spots and should not look dry or wilted. Avoid prepackaged spinach that has condensation. "Baby spinach" is picked sooner and will have smaller, more tender leaves, while mature spinach will be larger. Both taste about the same and will purée equally well.

Source Often plentiful and available at grocery stores year-round, but farmers' markets or produce stands may have fresher spinach. Peak harvest is from August to October or early spring, depending on the area.

Short-Term Storage Store unwashed in a perforated plastic bag in the vegetable crisper of the refrigerator for up to five days.

Long-Term Storage Wash, blanch, and freeze whole in vacuum-sealed bags, or wash, dice completely, or purée, then place in vacuum-sealed bags, and freeze for up to 12 months.

Flavor Spinach is often described as having a mild, earthy, and slightly sweet flavor. It is one of the cruciferous vegetables that has sulfur-containing compounds that get stronger when chopped, cooked, or chewed, all of which release the compounds. This increases the smell and associated flavor, which can be unpleasant.

Texture Stems can be crunchy, but the leaves are softer. If it's not well-washed, it may have a gritty texture, and if overcooked, it will become limp and mushy.

Spices and Flavors that Disguise or Offset Bitterness

Garlic	Lemon juice
Pepper	Red pepper flakes
Nutmeg	

Nutritional Benefits Considered a superfood, Spinach is rich in vitamins A, C, & K; magnesium; iron; calcium; and antioxidants.

Sweet Potato

Selecting Sweet potatoes should have smooth skin with no bruises or soft spots and no sign of sprouting from the eyes. Small to medium-sized ones tend to have better flavor.

Source Often plentiful and available at grocery stores year-round, but farmers' markets or produce stands may have fresher sweet potatoes, which tend to be sweeter. Peak harvest is from August to November, depending on the area.

Short-Term Storage Do not refrigerate; store in a cool, dark, dry spot outside the fridge, like a cupboard or root cellar, for 2 to 3 months. It's best not to store in an enclosed space with onions.

Long-Term Storage Sweet potatoes can be frozen for long-term storage. Wash well and blanch or bake, then flash freeze before transferring to airtight freezer bags to store for 8 to 12 months. It is not recommended to freeze raw sweet potatoes.

Flavor Sweet potatoes have a mild, starchy flavor similar to potatoes, but have a sweeter, nutty-like taste.

Texture Cooked sweet potatoes have a soft, smooth texture.

Spices that Blend Well

Cinnamon	Nutmeg
Ginger	Cloves

Nutritional Benefits Rich in vitamins A & C, fiber, and antioxidants.

Swiss Chard

Selecting Swiss Chard is typically packaged in bunches. Choose ones with firm stalks and broad, dark green leaves. Avoid any that are wilted, discolored, or have black spots or holes.

Source Often plentiful and available at grocery stores year-round, though farmers' markets or produce stands may have fresher chard, which tends to be sweeter. Peak harvest is from July to August, depending on the area.

Short-Term Storage Store unwashed in a perforated plastic bag in the vegetable crisper of the refrigerator for up to five days.

Long-Term Storage Wash, blanch, and freeze whole in vacuum-sealed bags or wash, dice completely, or purée, then place in vacuum-sealed bags and freeze for up to 12 months.

Flavor Swiss chard leaves have a mild, earthy flavor. The flavor is similar to spinach and kale but less bitter. It becomes even more mild when cooked.

Texture Stems are crisp and crunchy; leaves are soft and have a nubby-like surface.

Spices and Flavors that Cut the Bitterness

Red Wine Vinegar	Garlic
Lemon Juice	Red Pepper Flakes

Nutritional Benefits Considered a superfood, Swiss Chard is rich in vitamins A, C, & K; magnesium; potassium; calcium; and antioxidants.

Tomato

Selecting Ripe tomatoes should have a rich, consistent color, usually deep orange or red, and feel firm but have a slight "give" when squeezed. If they feel hard, they haven't fully ripened. The skin should feel smooth and shiny, without any cracks, dark spots, bruises, or blemishes.

Source Readily available at grocery stores year-round, but farmers' markets or produce stands may have fresher options and a greater variety. Peak harvest is from August to October, depending on the area.

Short-Term Storage For fresh tomatoes not fully ripened (still light-colored or very firm), keep them at room temperature away from direct sunlight for 1 to 5 days while ripening. If ripened, store in the refrigerator, but not in the crisper drawer, for 2 to 3 days.

Long-Term Storage Tomatoes can be frozen whole (after washing and removing stem and core), blanched and chopped, or puréed in vacuum-sealed bags and frozen for up to 12 months.

Flavor Tomatoes are juicy when raw and have a sweet and sometimes tangy taste, but overall mild. They become even milder cooked.

Texture Raw tomatoes are juicy and can be crunchy. When cooked, they are soft.

Spices and Flavors that Blend Well

Garlic	Onion
Oregano	Red Pepper Flakes
Baking Soda or Lemon Juice to reduce the acidity	

Nutritional Benefits Tomatoes are a good source of vitamins C & K and potassium and are high in antioxidants.

Zucchini

Selecting Zucchini should feel firm and have a vibrant color, usually green, but it may be yellow or white. The skin should be smooth and shiny without wrinkles or pits and not have any soft spots. Smaller zucchinis—about 6 to 8 inches long—are considered to have the best flavor and are easier to slice. Larger zucchini will have less flavor. Larger seeds that are easy to remove have equal nutritional value to smaller ones.

Source Readily available at grocery stores year-round, but farmers' markets or produce stands may have fresher options and a greater variety. They can be available any time of year, only taking 60 days from planting to maturity.

Short-Term Storage Store whole, dry, and unwashed in an open-ended paper bag or a plastic bag with a dry paper towel in the refrigeration crisper drawer. Will stay fresh for up to two weeks. If cut, store it in a sealed container in the refrigerator for up to five days.

Long-Term Storage Shred, drain excess moisture, then place in vacuum-sealed bags and freeze for up to 12 months. When it thaws, it will have a lot of moisture so be prepared to drain it but save the nutrition-packed juice!

Flavor Zucchini is very mild and slightly sweet, sometimes nearly tasteless.

Texture Raw zucchini is crisp and juicy. When cooked, it becomes very soft and blends easily with other food. It can have the texture of cooked spaghetti if cut into thin strips.

Spices and Flavors that Blend Well or Disguise
Zucchini blends well with virtually any spice.

Nutritional Benefits Zucchini is a good source of vitamins A, B6, C, & K; folate; and manganese.

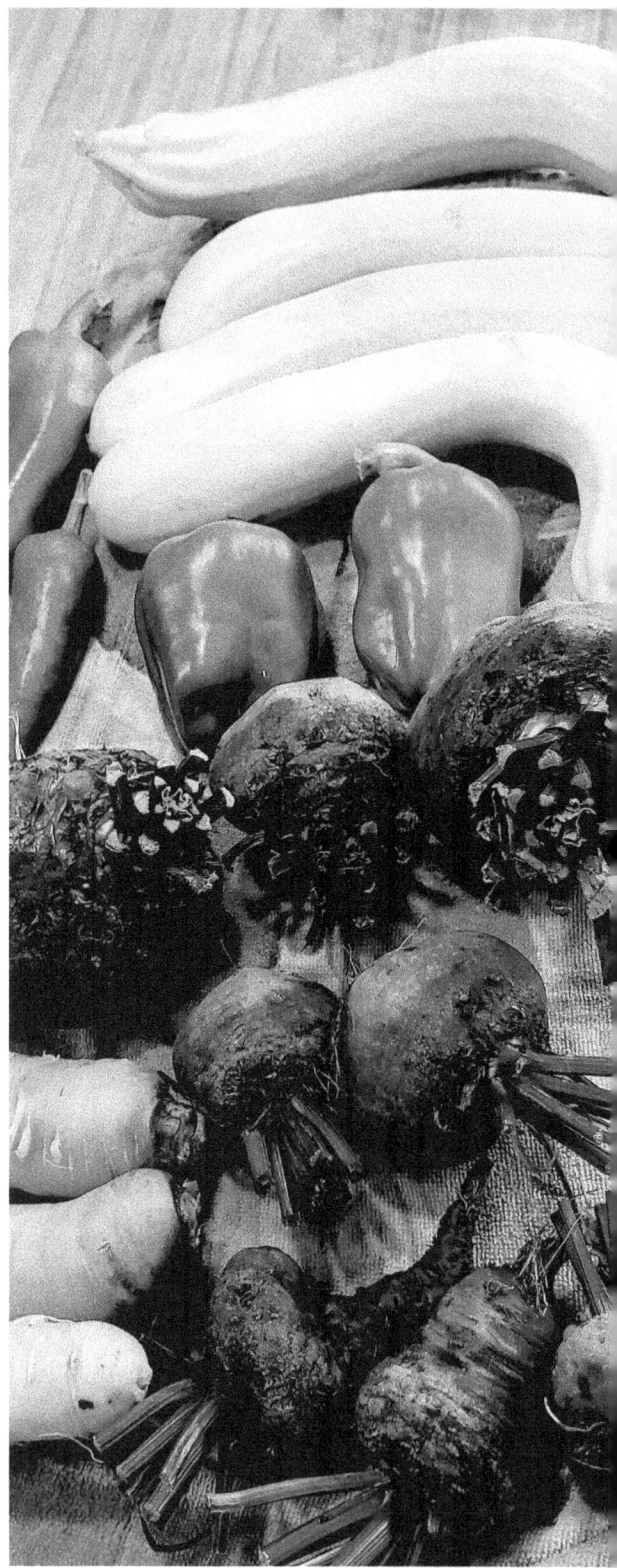

Using Top-Quality Weapons

Useful Equipment and Kitchen Tools

Knives

Chef's knife A chef's knife might be the most useful kitchen tool and can be used for 75% of all your vegetable cutting, chopping, and even dicing needs. The blade ranges from 6 inches to 12 inches and has a pointed, triangular blade. It is slightly curved, allowing you to press the tip into the cutting board while rocking the knife and using the blade heel to quickly chop and dice.

Cleaver A cleaver is usually associated with a butcher shop, but is excellent for slicing tougher vegetables such as kohlrabi, pumpkin, or squash. It has the added benefit of having a wide, flat blade that makes it easy to use the blunt edge (as opposed to the sharp edge) as a scraper to transfer chopped veggies into a food processor or pan.

Santoku Knife Similar to a chef's knife but smaller, usually with a 5-inch to 7-inch blade, a santoku knife is useful for dicing and mincing. It doesn't have the sharp tip and curved blade of a chef's knife, so it is not as versatile for chopping. But it is ideal for veggies with higher water content like zucchini.

Utility Knife This general-use knife is larger than a paring knife and smaller than the chef's knife, with a blade ranging from 4 inches to 9 inches. It can have a serrated edge, which is perfect for cutting tomatoes and other soft vegetables.

Paring Knife This basic, small knife has a sharp, non-serrated blade around 2½ inches to 4 inches long. It is excellent for peeling roasted beets, coring vegetables, and mincing small amounts.

Cutting Board

A cutting board is important for your cutting and chopping tasks. Using a quality cutting board will protect not only your knives but also the surface of counters and tabletops while providing a more stable cutting surface, making it easier to clean up afterward, and also preventing cross-contamination in the kitchen. Cross-contamination occurs when bacteria or viruses are transferred from one surface to another, which can lead to food poisoning. To prevent this, raw and cooked foods should remain separate, and good practices such as thorough hand-washing and properly cleaning surfaces and utensils should be followed.

Plastic cutting boards are common because they're inexpensive and easy to clean, plus widely available. Wood is a great choice and has the advantage of being easier on knives, so you'll have to sharpen less. Wood tends to harbor fewer bacteria, and some varieties, such as maple, walnut, and cherry, have natural antibacterial properties that may be retained through the cutting board manufacturing process. Choose the one that best suits your needs and preferences.

Vegetable Peeler

A good vegetable peeler will allow you to easily remove the outer skin or peel of vegetables. Peeling can be necessary because some vegetables have very tough skins; it also helps eliminate some of the more unpleasant flavors, plus help remove residual pesticides and fertilizers. However, many vegetables will have a high concentration of nutrients in the skin, so it may not always be advisable to peel them completely. Some examples where keeping the skin is beneficial are carrots, potatoes, zucchini, and bell peppers.

There are several types of peelers available, and there's no right or wrong choice. Select one that is comfortable, easy to clean, durable, and within your budget. You can check out second-hand stores for ones with enough residual life. There are many styles on the market that you can consider.

Swivel Swivel peelers function as the name indicates—they swivel to make it easier to follow the contours of irregular-shaped vegetables. Many swivel peelers allow you to change blade heads. They're great for potatoes, beets, and zucchini.

Y-Shape Also named for its primary design feature, this one has a straight fixed blade secured to the frame on either side. The frame is a "Y" shape, with the handle perpendicular to the blade. These are made for comfort, grip, and stability. They also cut in both directions, which allows you to work faster, so they're a great choice for carrots. They also work well for potatoes, beets, and zucchini.

Straight One of the most common and inexpensive peelers. The straight, simple design is practical and easy to use for basic peeling and tends to be easier to use for thin vegetables. They're perfect for straight, consistent veggies such as carrots and zucchini.

Serrated Sharp teeth on a serrated peeler will help grip tougher or smoother skin veggies. This is perfect for tomatoes and peppers.

Julienne Julienne peelers can be a great choice for certain vegetables, especially ones you want to create small strips out of. They're great for carrots and kohlrabi, to have a different small portion as an option to riced or diced.

Rotary Rotary peelers are good for basic peeling. They rotate in an enclosed circle as opposed to swiveling. They often also come with interchangeable blades so you can have basic, julienne, and serrated options just by changing the blade.

Grater A hand tool with a series of small holes used to wear down vegetables into small pieces. There are several types including box graters, rotary, rasp, and paddle graters. This tool is also used to zest fruit and grate cheese or spices like ginger and cinnamon.

Spiral Cutter A specialized cutter to create long, thin ribbons of vegetables like zucchini, carrot, sweet potatoes, and potatoes. It's great for vegetables as a pasta substitute or potato and sweet potato spirals for frying.

Vegetable Chopper A vegetable chopper is a smaller, scaled-down, and less expensive option for a food processor. Most have a single blade and typically do a great job of chopping, mincing, and puréeing smaller amounts. Their capacity ranges from 3 to 5 cups, depending on the model. Several options are available, both manual and electric. Choose the one that best suits your veggie goals, kitchen space, and budget.

- A manual cutter/chopper/dicer can do a good job of getting vegetables to about ½-inch size, sometimes smaller, depending on the unit.
- A rotary handle is another design for a manual vegetable shredder that can also slice, and grate.
- An electric vegetable chopper is an economical and readily available option. Choose one with multiple setting options such as purée, blend, or emulsify.

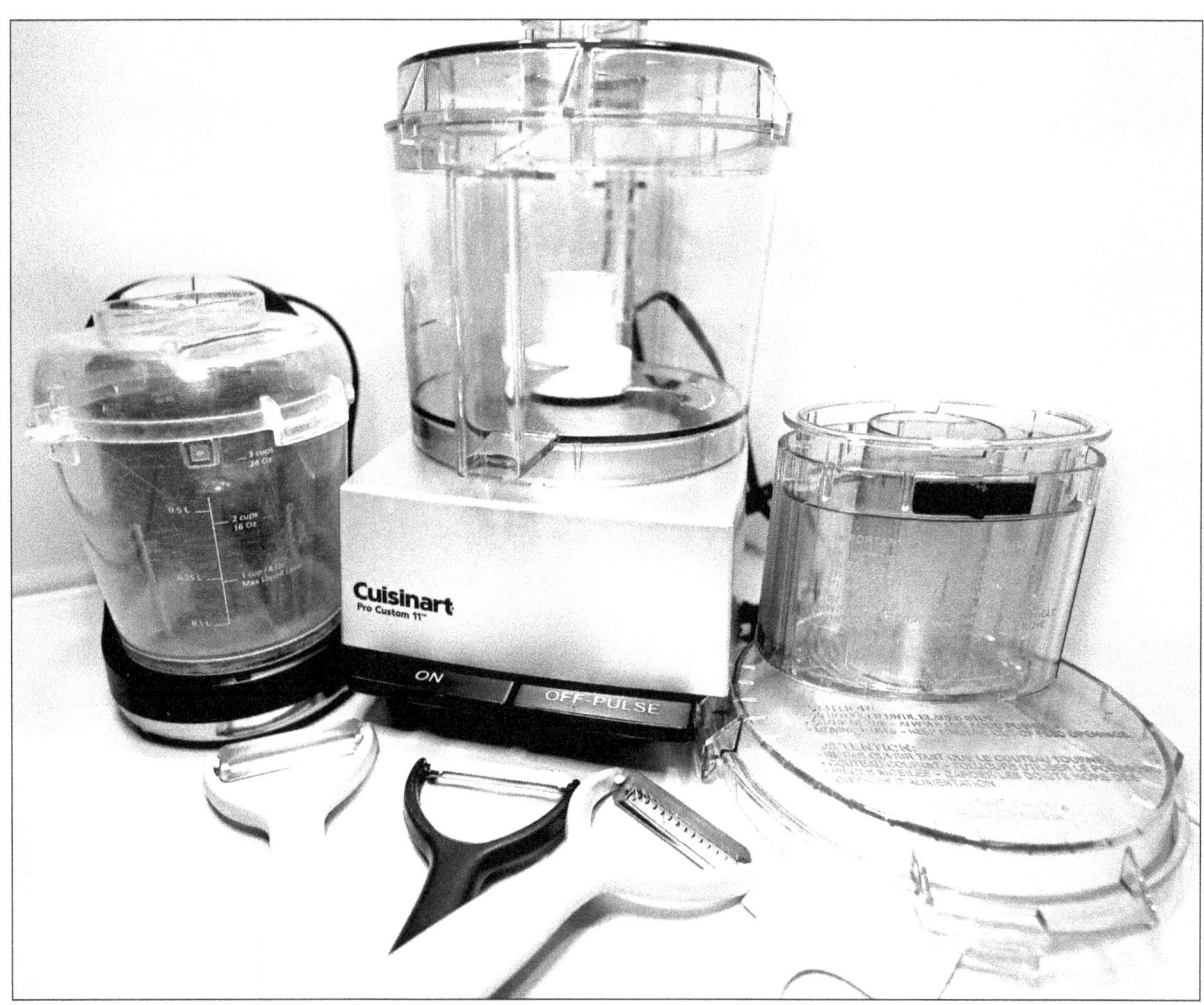

Food Processor A food processor is like a chopper, but larger, more powerful, and more flexible. Food processors have multiple blades that allow you to slice, shred, dice, grate, chop, and purée. Typically, extra power allows you to dice and grate more finely, which results in smoother purées. The design also has a feeder tube so that the machine can continue running as you add vegetables or liquid. It saves time and tends to be less messy, especially if you're processing large amounts.

Juicer A manual or electric juicer presses, grinds, or squeezes juice from vegetables. It is a great tool to use for making smoothies and creating juice for jelly or a liquid for cooking. The relative advantage juicers have over food processors or blenders is that they're designed to filter the juice from the pulp and fibrous parts of the vegetable. If you juice vegetables, save the pulp in freezer bags to add to soups, stews, and hot pot dishes.

Mesh Strainer Small kitchen tool to strain the juice and remove the pulp from puréed vegetables. An inexpensive item available in various sizes, this is excellent for cauliflower rice, zucchini, and puréed vegetables like beets, spinach, and kale.

Varying Methods of Attack

Terms

Blend Combine ingredients using a spoon or electric mixer until a consistent texture and color is achieved.

Chop Using a chef's knife, cut into small irregular-sized pieces, about ¼-inch long, or bite-sized. *Finely Chop* refers to taking it down to about ⅛-inch pieces, which do not have to be uniform.

Core Use a paring knife to remove the hard center of the vegetable, often the part with seeds.

Dice Using a chef's knife, cut into uniform small pieces, about ¼-inch, usually small squares. Finely Dice refers to taking it down to about ⅛-inch pieces, still of uniform shape.

Fold Gently mix ingredients using a spatula or spoon, bringing a portion of batter from the bowl's bottom to the top, to add a heavier ingredient without overmixing.

Grate Using a kitchen tool with holes, rub the vegetable against the surface to create small pieces or shavings.

Juice To squeeze, press, or grind vegetables using a manual or electric appliance until a liquid is produced.

Julienne Using a santoku knife, utility knife, or peeler to trim vegetables into thin, uniform, matchstick-like strips.

Mince The smallest measure of chopping vegetables, best done with an electric chopper or food processor. Mincing is one step away from purée and can look like coarse paste.

Mix Combine two or more ingredients with a whisk, spoon, or mixer until all ingredients are incorporated and thoroughly combined.

Peel Using a vegetable peeler or paring knife to remove the outer layer or skin of the vegetable.

Purée Using a blender, chopper, or food processor, to blend chopped vegetables into a thick liquid, keeping the pulp.

Rice Using a food processor to process uncooked dry vegetables down to the smallest piece. Dryer raw vegetables such as Brussels sprouts, broccoli, and cauliflower resist purée and will be processed to a rice-like size and consistency unless cooked first.

I use this term frequently! The correct and official definition is to force food through a food mill or ricer to produce a consistency smoother than mashing but coarser than purée. Once the term "riced cauliflower" became popular, and I realized vegetables could be broken down to near dust, I immediately applied the word and idea to as many vegetables as possible.

Shred Using a grater or food processor to create thin, long strips.

Slice Using a chef's knife to cut vegetables into thin, flat pieces.

Stir To mix ingredients or liquid using a spoon in a circular motion for even distribution and/or to prevent burning.

Whisk To blend quickly and completely using a metal or plastic whisk.

Be Versatile and Agile

Seasoning & Cooking Tips

The whole point of this cookbook is to provide you with recipes you'll love to eat that incorporate healthy vegetables without highlighting their flavor. So, start with your own favorite recipes or use the flavors you like and incorporate the vegetables. You can use balsamic vinegar, Parmesan cheese, garlic powder, and onion powder on mild vegetables such as asparagus or zucchini to suppress their taste.

Strong flavors like chili powder or hot sauce often overpower vegetables like sweet potato, cauliflower, and carrots.

The strongest tasting, and often bitter, ones like kale and spinach are best incorporated into complex recipes that have lots of seasonings and ingredients.

Some, like kohlrabi, sweet potatoes, or carrots, can easily blend with sweeter flavors like honey, almond, apple, and maple syrup. Don't be afraid to experiment. If you're like me and already dislike them, it usually can't make them any worse.

Last but not least, ordinary salt will often minimize the bitterness or unpleasant flavor in many vegetables.

Preserve the Nutrients

Keep vegetables fresh and raw before dicing, mincing, or puréeing, and add directly into recipes to incorporate the nutrients into the dish you're preparing. Avoid boiling because the nutrients end up in the water, and many vegetables will get mushy and even less appealing. Baking, steaming, or microwaving will cook or soften before puréeing while preserving most of the nutrients.

Steam in the microwave: Clean, peel, and chop veggies. Place in a microwave-safe bowl with 2–3 tablespoons of water. Cover the bowl, and microwave on high for 3 to 4 minutes.

Steam on the stovetop without a steamer basket: Take up to a ½ inch of water in a pan. Place four small balls of aluminum foil in the water at the bottom of the pan and keep a heat-proof plate on the balls so that it does not touch the bottom of the pan. Cover the pan and set on high heat until boiling. Clean, peel, and chop the veggies while the water is heating. Once the water boils, carefully add the chopped vegetables to the pan, then cover and steam for 7–9 minutes or until tender.

Avoid Flatulence

Cruciferous vegetables such as cauliflower, broccoli, Brussels sprouts, cabbage, kale, and kohlrabi have sulfur-containing compounds that get stronger when cooked, causing an odor many people find unpleasant. Chopping, cooking, or chewing releases the compound, thereby increasing the smell and associated flavor. For some people, this also causes flatulence. Certain spices may help counteract the gas and mask the flavor/smell.

- Use turmeric, cumin, fennel, coriander, garlic powder, or ginger in savory recipes.
- Use ginger, cinnamon, cloves, mint, or cardamom in sweeter recipes.

Don't Plan Everything in Detail

Let yourself have fun with recipes and try new combinations. Experiment but keep notes. Nothing's worse than a fantastic creation you cannot replicate.

- Use **puréed beets** in place of vegetable or canola oil. It's an easy 1:1 ratio, but keep in mind that beet may change the color of your dish.
- Add **cauliflower** or **zucchini** juice to a smoothie. You'll create juice when you **rice cauliflower** and when you **shred zucchini.** Keep this in a small jar (stored separately) to either add to smoothies or to zing up your water.

The Hidden Vegetables Cookbook

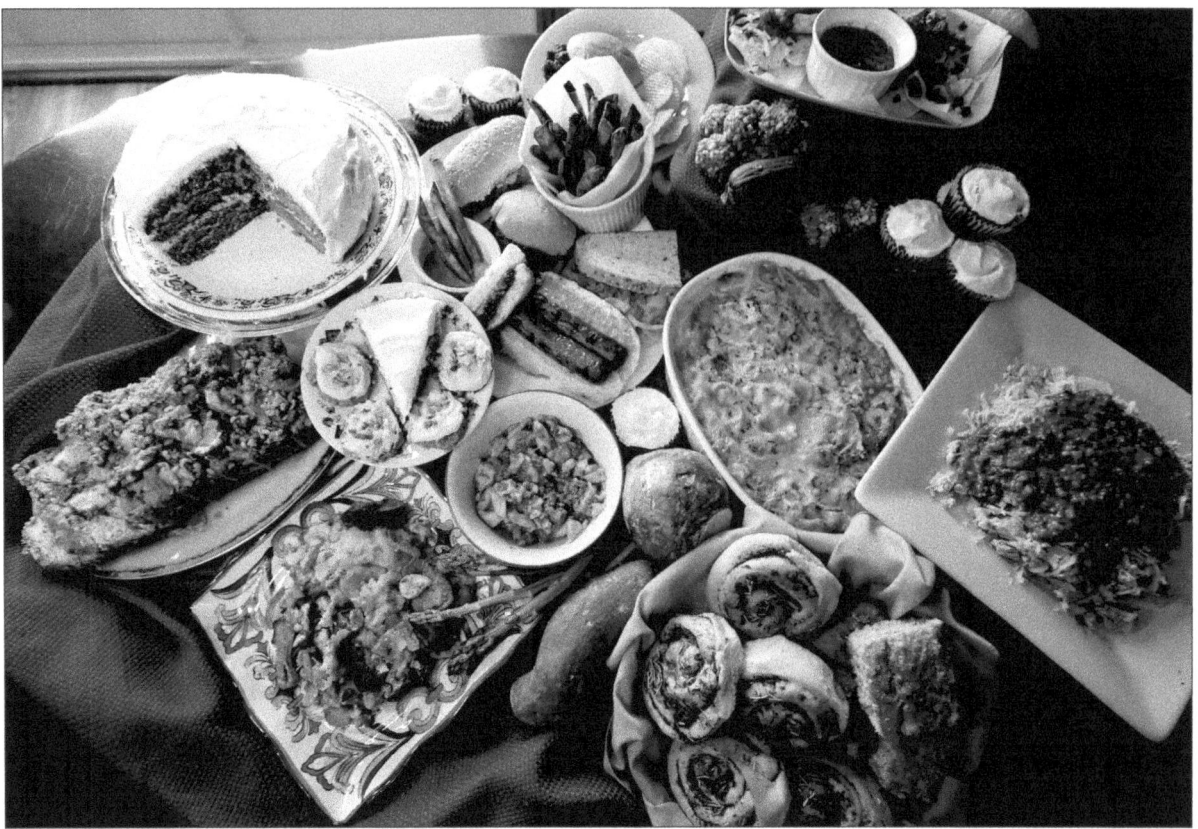

- Add **cauliflower juice** or **zucchini juice** to your morning oatmeal in place of water.

- Keep riced and chopped veggies in the freezer. Throw in a handful when you're preparing a dish. This strategy works for goulash, one-pot meals, and many crock-pot dishes. When lots of flavors are involved or slow cooking for a long time is required, smaller pieces of veggies will blend in, often becoming indistinguishable in flavor, although most of their nutrition will remain.

Be creative!
Add your notes here:

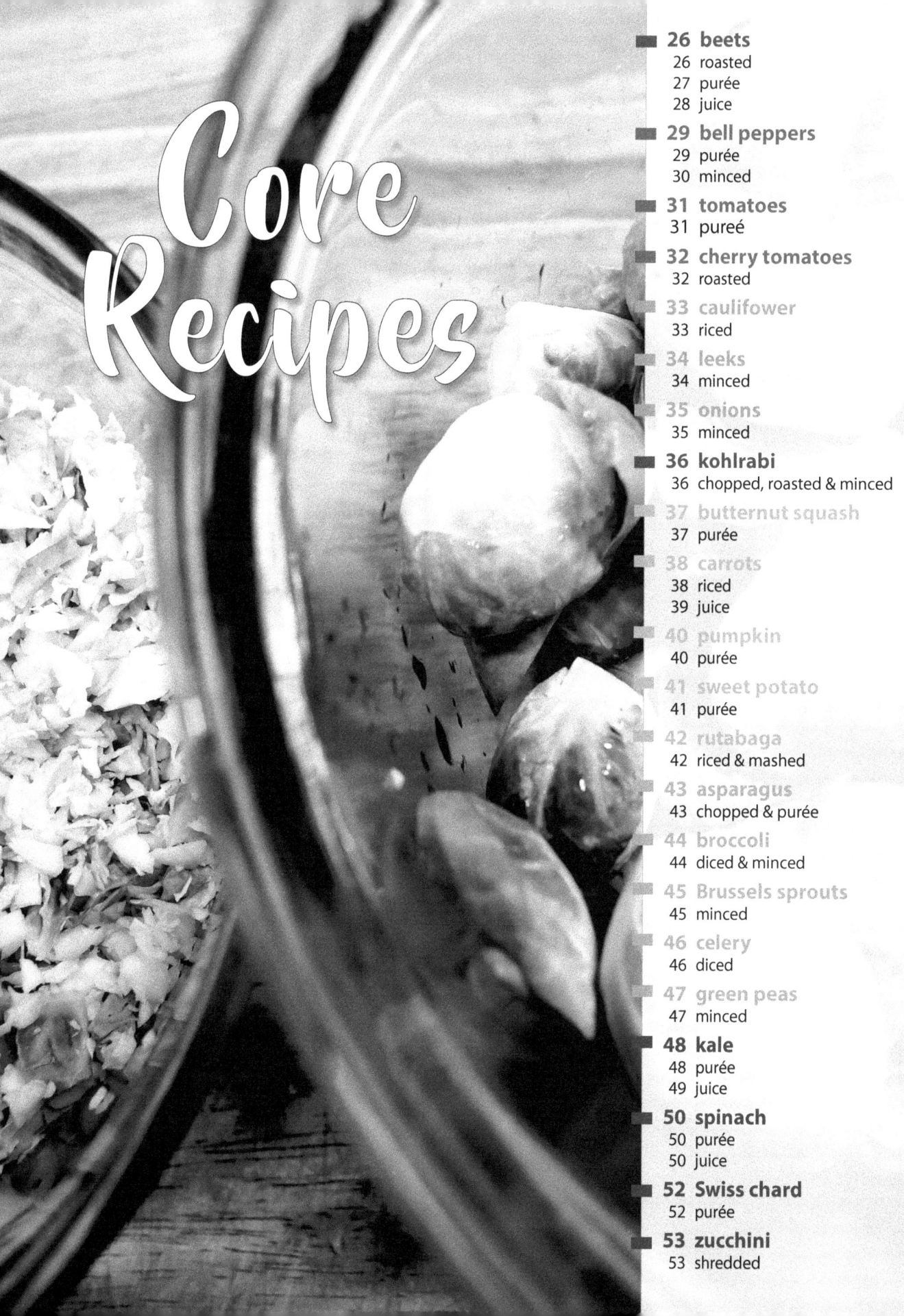

Core Recipes

- **26 beets**
  - 26 roasted
  - 27 purée
  - 28 juice
- **29 bell peppers**
  - 29 purée
  - 30 minced
- **31 tomatoes**
  - 31 pureé
- **32 cherry tomatoes**
  - 32 roasted
- **33 cauliflower**
  - 33 riced
- **34 leeks**
  - 34 minced
- **35 onions**
  - 35 minced
- **36 kohlrabi**
  - 36 chopped, roasted & minced
- **37 butternut squash**
  - 37 purée
- **38 carrots**
  - 38 riced
  - 39 juice
- **40 pumpkin**
  - 40 purée
- **41 sweet potato**
  - 41 purée
- **42 rutabaga**
  - 42 riced & mashed
- **43 asparagus**
  - 43 chopped & purée
- **44 broccoli**
  - 44 diced & minced
- **45 Brussels sprouts**
  - 45 minced
- **46 celery**
  - 46 diced
- **47 green peas**
  - 47 minced
- **48 kale**
  - 48 purée
  - 49 juice
- **50 spinach**
  - 50 purée
  - 50 juice
- **52 Swiss chard**
  - 52 purée
- **53 zucchini**
  - 53 shredded

beets: roasted

ingredients
Fresh beets (any variety)

directions
1. Preheat oven to 350 °F.
2. Trim green and root to about 1 inch.
3. Rinse away any dirt. Pat dry.
4. Brush skin with olive oil.
5. Wrap individually in foil and place on a baking sheet.
6. Bake for 50 to 60 minutes or until they are soft when poked with a knife.
7. Remove from oven, unwrap, and discard foil.
8. Allow beets to cool before handling. Then, use a sharp knife to cut the coarse outer skin and peel it away.
9. Chop into 1-inch squares.
10. Use immediately or store in a refrigerator for 2 to 3 days.

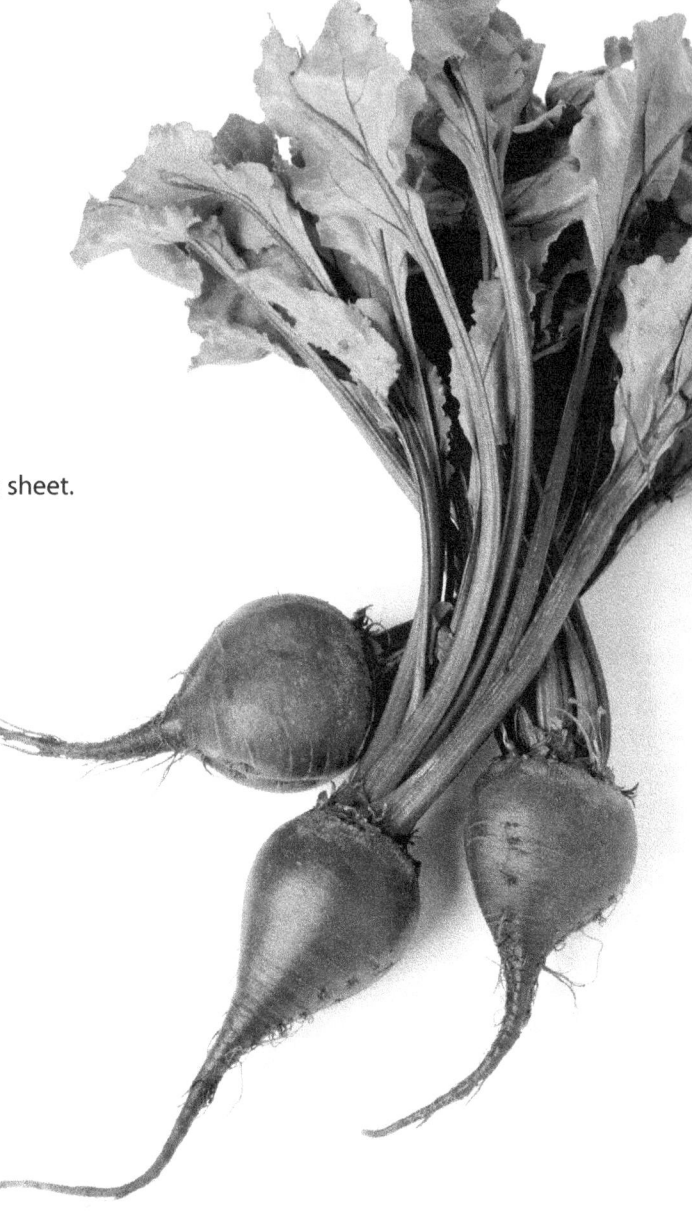

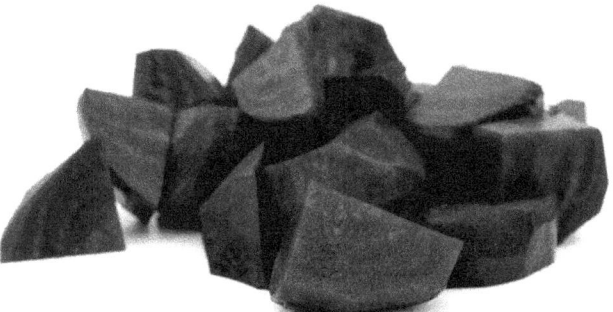

chopped roasted beets

---

from the Health and Wellness Coach

Nutrients Folate, manganese, fiber, nitrates

Benefits Improve blood flow, support liver function, and may enhance endurance

Fun Fact Beet juice is popular with athletes for its stamina-boosting powers

beets: purée

yield
Two large beets (any variety) will yield approximately one cup of beet purée.

directions
1. Preheat oven to 350°F.
2. Trim green and root to about 1inch.
3. Rinse away any dirt. Pat dry.
4. Brush skin with olive oil.
5. Wrap individually in foil and place on a baking sheet.
6. Bake for 50 to 60 minutes or until they are soft when poked with a knife.
7. Remove from oven, unwrap, and discard foil.
8. Allow beets to cool before handling. Then, use a sharp knife to cut the coarse outer skin and peel it away.
9. Chop into 1- to 2-inch pieces.
10. Using a blender or food processor, mix on high until smooth to create a thick purée.
11. Use immediately or store in a refrigerator for 2 to 3 days. For longer-term storage, freeze in portions.

freezing
12. Pour the purée into ice cube trays and freeze until solid.
13. Transfer to freezer-safe bags. Remove as much air as possible and seal.
14. Measure out individual cubes for recipes: Most ice cube trays have a 1-inch well that will hold about 1 ounce of liquid.
    8 cubes = 1 cup;
    4 cubes = ½ cup;
    2 cubes = ¼ cup
15. Properly sealed purée will stay fresh for 6 to 8 months.

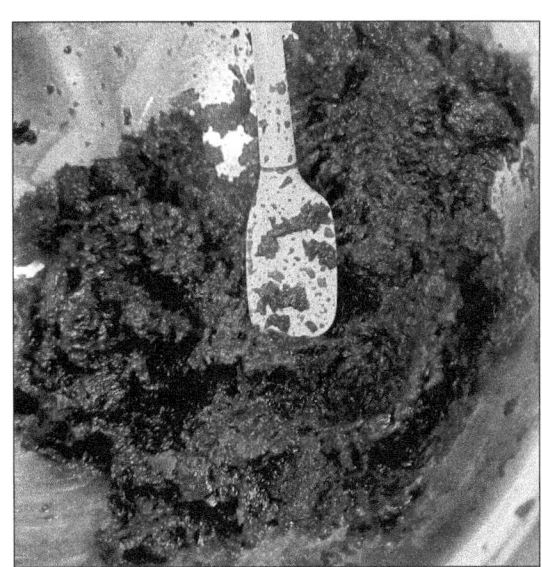

beet purée

beet juice
(without a juicer)

ingredients
Fresh beets (any variety)

directions
Follow directions for **Beet Purée** from page 27:

1. Preheat oven to 350°F.
2. Trim green and root to about 1 inch.
3. Rinse away any dirt. Pat dry.
4. Brush skin with olive oil.
5. Wrap individually in foil and place on a baking sheet.
6. Bake for 50 to 60 minutes or until they are soft when poked with a knife.
7. Remove from oven, unwrap, and discard foil.
8. Allow beets to cool before handling. Then, use a sharp knife to cut the coarse outer skin and peel it away.
9. Chop into 1- to 2-inch pieces.
10. Using a blender or food processor, mix on high until smooth to create a thick purée.
11. Strain through a colander lined with cheesecloth to separate juice from pulp.
12. Add the pulp back to the purée to keep for recipes.

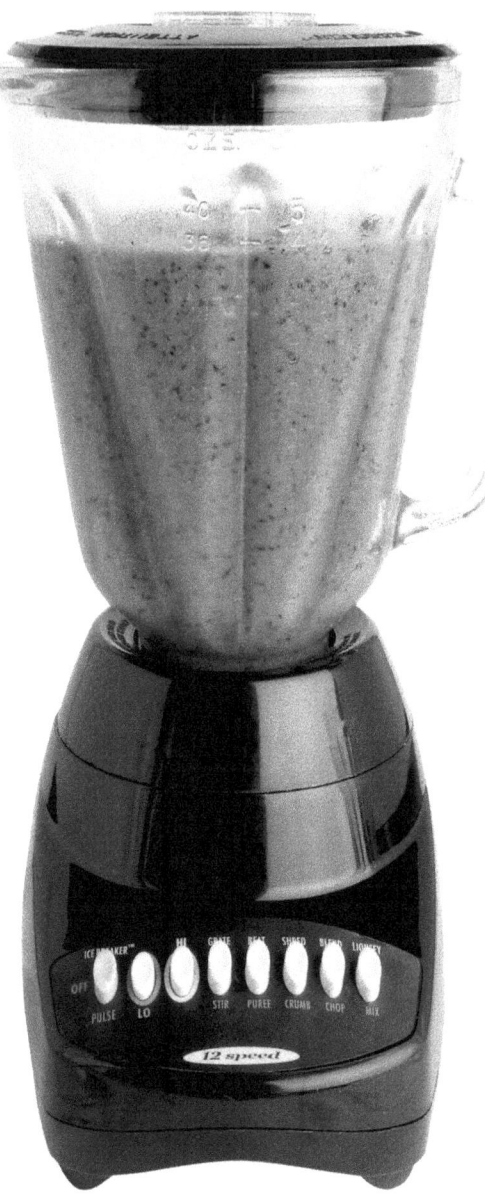

from the **Health and Wellness Coach**

Nutrients Folate, manganese, fiber, nitrates

Benefits Improve blood flow, support liver function, and may enhance endurance

Fun Fact Beet juice is popular with athletes for its stamina-boosting powers

bell peppers: purée

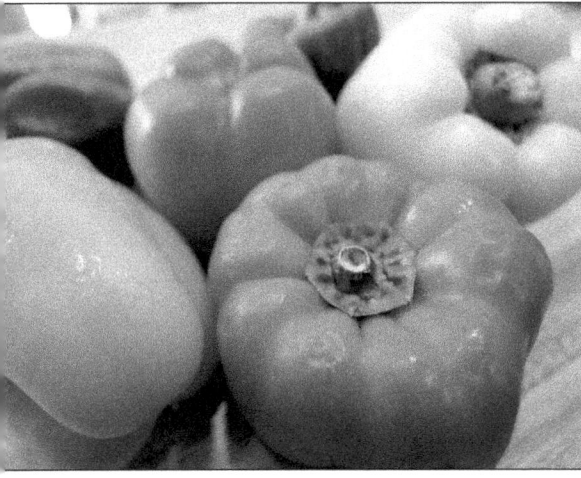

yield
Two large bell peppers (any variety) will yield approximately one cup of bell pepper purée.

directions
1. Preheat oven to 450°F.
2. Wash peppers by rinsing them under cold water to remove any dirt or debris.
3. Cut off the stem and top, then slice in half.
4. Use a paper towel to pat dry.
5. Line a baking sheet with parchment paper.
6. Lay sliced peppers skin side up on the prepared baking sheet.
7. Bake for 20 minutes, turn, then bake an additional 20 minutes.
8. Remove from oven and cool.
9. Peel off the outer skin; remove the seeds and inner membrane, and discard.
10. Place the roasted peppers in a food processor and pulse on high until puréed.
11. Pack into ice cube trays and freeze until solid.
12. Transfer to freezer-safe bags. Remove as much air as possible and seal.
13. Measure out individual cubes for recipes:
    Most ice cube trays have a 1-inch well that will hold about 1 ounce of liquid.
    - 8 cubes = 1 cup;
    - 4 cubes = ½ cup;
    - 2 cubes = ¼ cup
14. Properly sealed purée will stay fresh for 6 to 8 months.

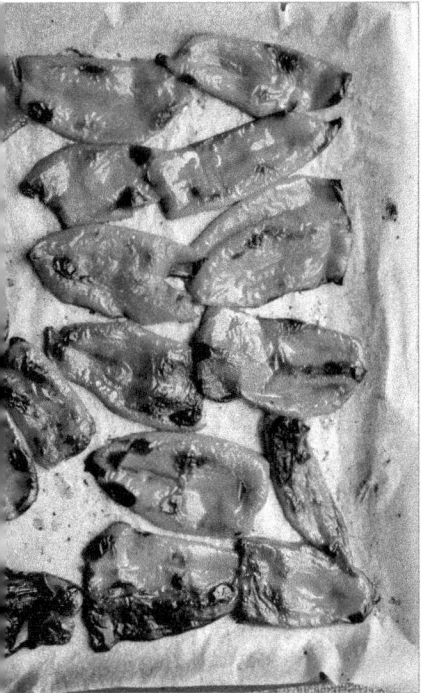

pan of roasted red peppers

---

from the **Health and Wellness Coach**

Nutrients Vitamins A, C, B6, folate, fiber

Benefits Help with immune support, eye health, and inflammation reduction

Fun Fact Red bell peppers have more vitamin C than an orange—seriously

bell peppers: minced

yield
One large bell pepper (any variety) will yield approximately one cup of diced bell pepper.

directions
1. Wash peppers by rinsing them under cold water to remove any dirt or debris.
2. Cut off the stem and top, then slice in half.
3. Remove the seeds and inner membrane.
4. Use a paper towel to pat dry.
5. Cut the peppers into strips or chunks of up to 3 inches.
6. Spread the prepared peppers in a single layer on a baking sheet or tray lined with parchment paper. Place the tray in the freezer for about an hour to allow the peppers to freeze solid.
7. Remove from the tray and place the frozen pieces in freezer-safe bags. Remove as much air as possible and seal. Properly sealed, the peppers will stay fresh for 6 to 8 months.
8. To use, remove frozen pieces and place them in a food processor to mince. They can be processed easily. The pieces may retain some ice crystals, which is fine.
9. Measure out for the recipe once the peppers are minced.

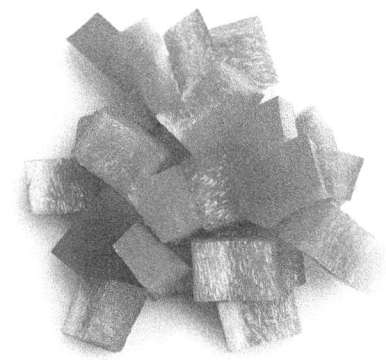

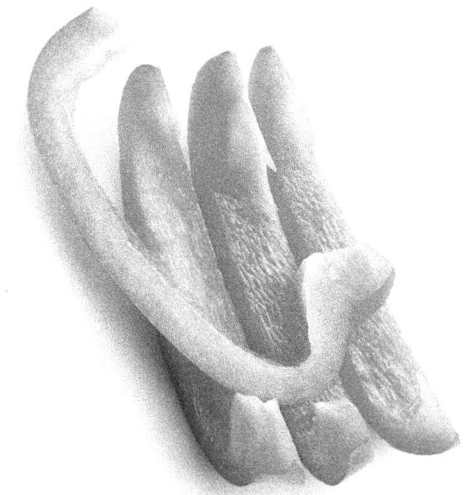

from the **Health and Wellness Coach**

Nutrients Vitamins A, C, B6, folate, fiber

Benefits Help with immune support, eye health, and inflammation reduction

Fun Fact Red bell peppers have more vitamin C than an orange—seriously

tomato: purée

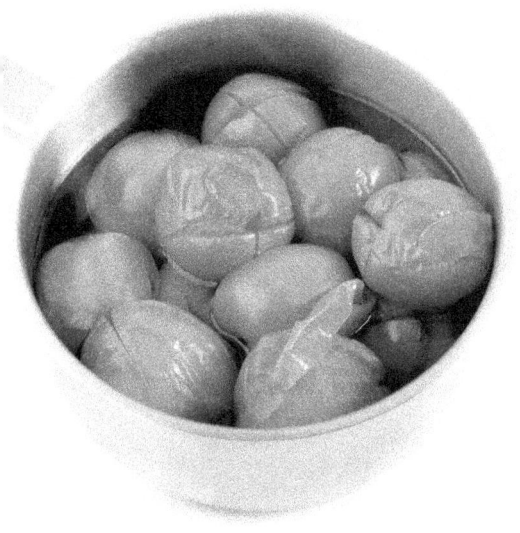

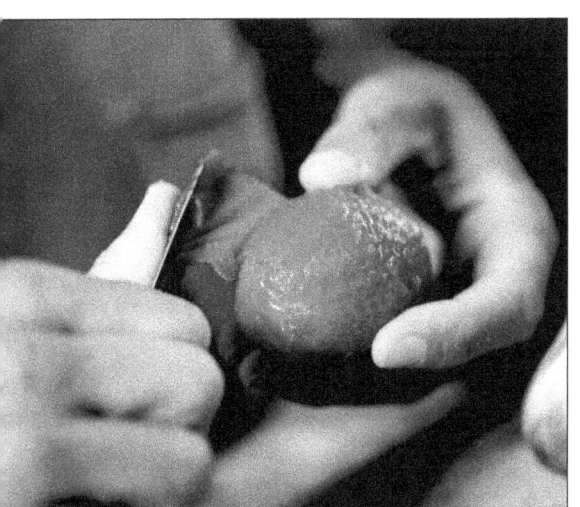

yield
Two pounds tomatoes (any variety) will yield approximately one cup of tomato purée.

directions
1. Rinse tomatoes using cold running water to remove dirt and debris.
2. With a sharp knife, pierce the skin at the bottom, making a cut about ½ inch long. Make a second cut across the first, forming an "X." Continue until all the tomatoes are cut.
3. Prepare a large bowl of ice water and set aside.
4. In a large stockpot, bring 4 quarts of water to a boil.
5. Place the tomatoes in the boiling water for 30 seconds to one minute, until the skin starts to split around the cuts. You may need to do this in batches if you are processing more than a dozen tomatoes.
6. Transfer the tomatoes from the boiling water to the ice water.
7. Once cool to the touch, peel off the skin and place the skinned tomatoes in a clean bowl. Discard skins.
8. Using a cutting board, cut each skinned tomato in half; remove the seeds and surrounding gel with a spoon or your fingers and discard. After the seeds are removed, roughly chop the tomatoes and place them in a stockpot. Do not add any additional liquid.
9. Simmer over medium heat until softened.
10. Transfer to a blender or food processor and pulse until the desired purée consistency is reached.
11. Use immediately or refrigerate for 2 to 3 days. For longer-term storage, freeze in portions.

freezing
1. Pour into ice cube trays and freeze until solid.
2. Transfer to freezer-safe bags. Remove as much air as possible and seal.
3. Measure out individual cubes for recipes: Most ice cube trays have a 1-inch well that will hold about 1 ounce of liquid.
   - 8 cubes = 1 cup;
   - 4 cubes = ½ cup;
   - 2 cubes = ¼ cup
4. Properly sealed, purée will stay fresh for 6 to 8 months.

---

from the Health and Wellness Coach

Nutrients Lycopene, vitamin C, potassium, folate

Benefits Good for heart health and skin; may protect against sunburn

Fun Fact Treated as a veggie, tomatoes are technically fruits—and were once considered poisonous!

cherry tomatoes: roasted

ingredients
2 tablespoons of olive oil

1 teaspoon minced garlic

¼ teaspoon red pepper

½ teaspoon salt

½ teaspoon pepper

cooking spray

directions
1. Preheat the oven to 400°F.
2. Line a sheet pan with parchment paper.
3. In a medium bowl, mix olive oil, garlic, red pepper, salt, and pepper.
4. Cut cherry tomatoes in half. Toss in olive oil mixture.
5. Lay coated tomatoes on the parchment in a single layer.
6. Bake for 25 minutes.
7. Remove from oven immediately and transfer to fresh parchment paper to dry.
8. Reset oven to 200°F and place the fresh tray in the oven for 90 minutes.
9. Use immediately or store in an airtight container in the refrigerator for 1 to 2 days.
10. For longer-term storage, spread the roasted tomatoes in a single layer on a baking sheet or tray lined with parchment paper.
11. Place the tray in the freezer for about an hour to allow the tomatoes to freeze solid.
12. Remove from the tray and place the frozen tomatoes in freezer-safe bags. Remove as much air as possible and seal. Properly sealed, tomatoes will stay fresh for 6 to 8 months.
13. To use in recipes, remove the frozen pieces and dice them in a food processor or use whole.

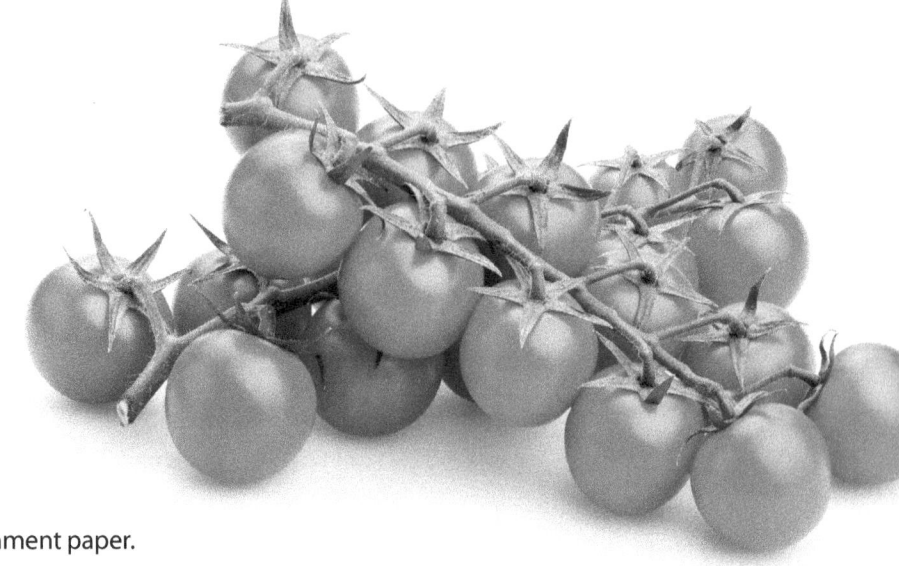

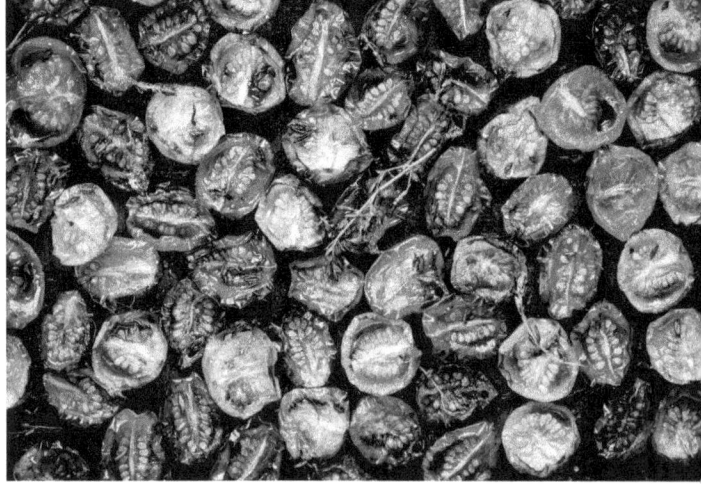

from the Health and Wellness Coach

Nutrients Lycopene, vitamin C, potassium, folate

Benefits Good for heart health and skin; may protect against sunburn

Fun Fact Treated as a veggie, tomatoes are technically fruits—and were once considered poisonous!

cauliflower flour
(riced cauliflower)

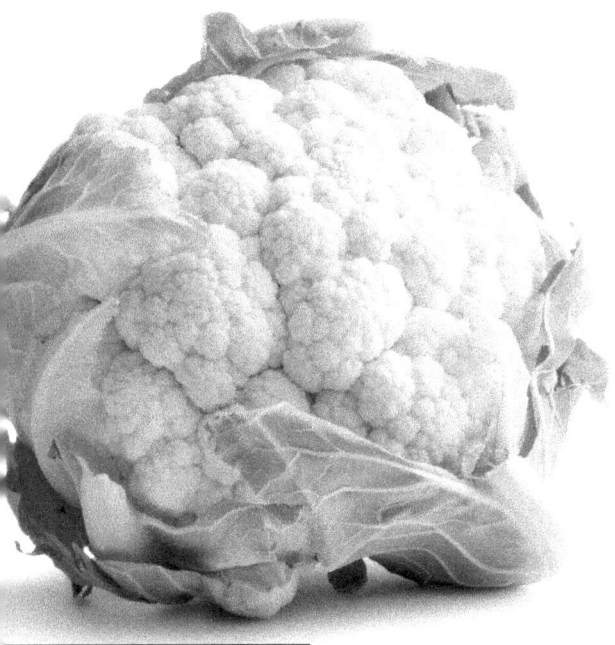

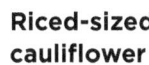

Riced-sized cauliflower

Squeezing riced, cooked, cooled cauliflower

yield

One pound (usually 1 head) of cauliflower florets will yield approximately four cups of riced cauliflower.

directions

1. Preheat oven to 400°F.

2. Cut off the base of the cauliflower and chop into small florets.

3. Place inside a food processor in batches, pulsing to reduce the cauliflower to the size and consistency of rice.

4. Pack the riced cauliflower in a glass baking dish and spread to distribute evenly. Bake for 15 minutes.

5. Remove from the oven and cool.

6. Spoon or scrape the purée onto a flour sack towel or a fine-weave cheesecloth and wrap tightly.

7. Squeeze the liquid out of the cauliflower over a measuring cup.
   - On average, every ½ pound of florets pulsed 4 to 5 times will yield about 2 cups of riced cauliflower.
   - The cheesecloth step should help to squeeze about ½ cup of liquid from the riced cauliflower.

8. Store the cauliflower water in a covered jar in the refrigerator. See page 54 for uses for the saved water.

9. Riced cauliflower can be stored in the refrigerator for 3 to 4 days.

10. For longer-term storage, transfer to freezer-safe bags. Remove as much air as possible, flatten, and seal. Riced cauliflower will stay fresh in the freezer for up to 8–12 months.

11. Remove from freezer and measure out portions for recipes as needed.

---

from the **Health and Wellness Coach**

Nutrients Vitamin C, K, folate, fiber

Benefits Supports detox and brain health, and is low-carb friendly

Fun Fact It's the chameleon of the veggie world—mashed, riced, even pizza crusted!

leeks: minced

yield
One leek will yield approximately one cup of minced leeks.

directions
1. To store leeks properly for freshness, keep them unwashed and untrimmed, wrapped loosely in a plastic bag or in a perforated plastic bag in the crisper drawer of your refrigerator, where they will last for 1 to 2 weeks.

2. When ready to use, lay on a cutting board.

3. Use a sharp knife to trim off the root end up to where individual circles separate into layers. Trim off the tougher, dark green top. Trim off any part that is withered, brown, or damaged.

4. Slice into one-inch sections, then slice each section in half.

5. Peel back the layers of each piece and wash well under cold running water.

6. Use a paper towel to remove excess water, then place the cleaned section in a food processor or blender.

7. Pulse to finely mince.

8. Use directly in recipes or store in a refrigerator in tightly sealed containers for up to 3 days.

9. For longer-term storage, place in freezer-safe bags. Remove as much air as possible and seal. Properly sealed, leeks will stay fresh for 6 to 8 months.

TIP: Freezing in storage bags after flattening to remove excess air will also help keep the package even and make the leeks break up for easier measurement and use in recipes.

---

from the **Health and Wellness Coach**

Nutrients Vitamin K, manganese, folate, iron

Benefits Support heart and bone health; prebiotic-rich

Fun Fact Leeks are celebrated in Wales and worn as a national symbol on St. David's Day

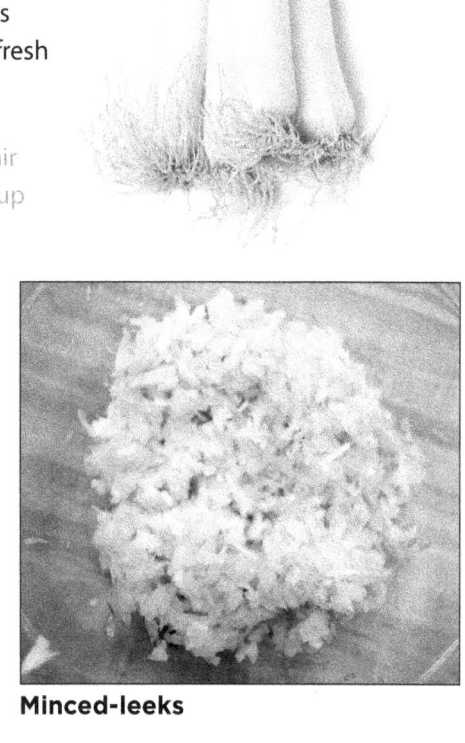

Minced-leeks

onion: minced

yield
One medium-sized onion (any color or variety) will yield approximately two cups of minced onion.

directions
1. Pull away and remove the dry outer layer.
2. Cut off the top and bottom ends.
3. Slice the onion into quarters.
4. Place the pieces in a food processor or blender.
5. Pulse to finely mince.
6. Use directly in recipes or store in a refrigerator in a tightly sealed container for 2 to 3 days.
7. For longer-term storage, place in freezer-safe bags. Remove as much air as possible and seal. Properly sealed onions will stay fresh for 6 to 8 months.

TIP: Freezing in storage bags and flattening to remove excess air will also help keep the package even and make the onions break up for easier measurement and use in recipes.

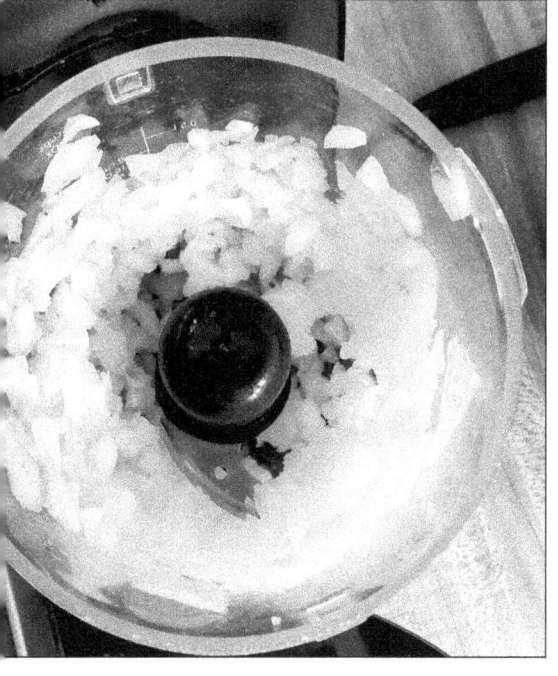

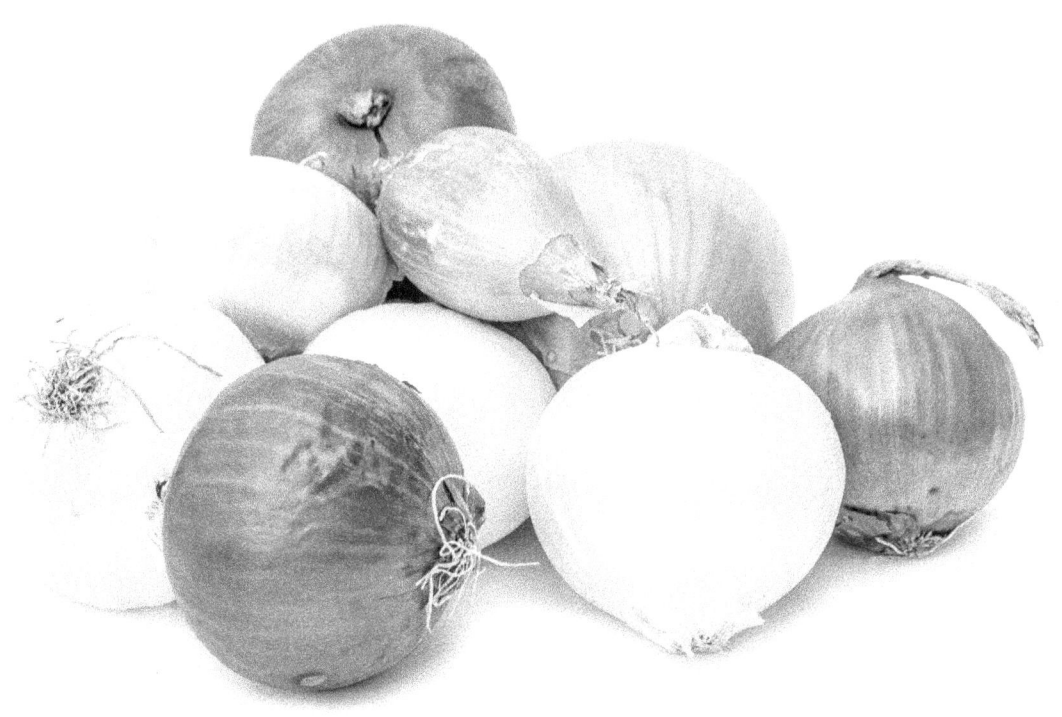

kohlrabi: chopped, roasted & minced

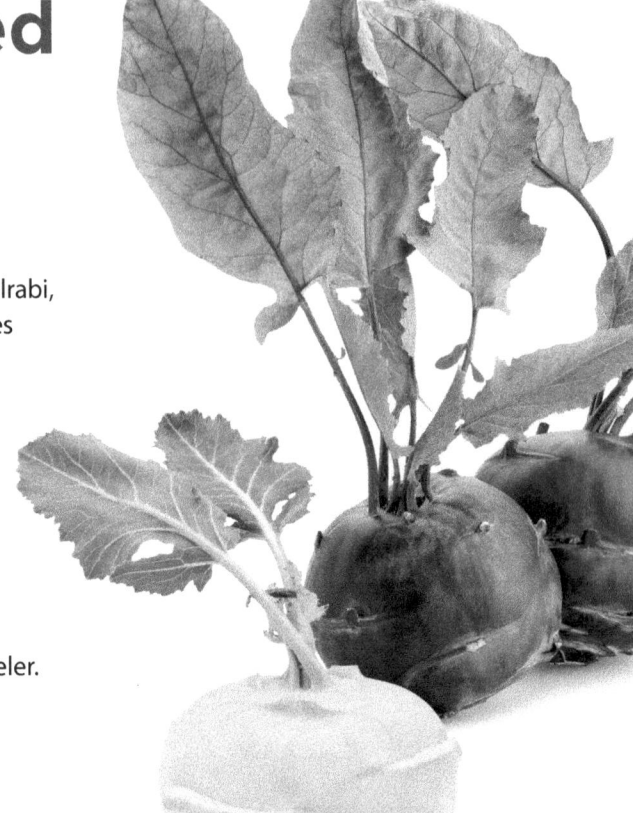

yield
One medium-sized kohlrabi (any variety) will yield approximately two cups of diced kohlrabi.

prepare
1. If the stems and leaves are still attached to the kohlrabi, cut them off. Set these aside; you can use the leaves later and purée them just like kale or spinach.
2. Cut the kohlrabi head in half down the center.
3. Slice into quarters.
4. Cut out the core by using the tip of your knife to cut at an angle through the core and discard the tough center part.
5. The skin contains nutritional benefit so remove only the toughest skin using a sharp vegetable peeler.
6. Roast or mince to use in recipes.

roast
1. Preheat oven to 425°F.
2. Roast the kohlrabi for 30 to 45 minutes until tender.
3. Remove from oven and place in a food processor. Add one tablespoon of water. Blend on the highest setting.
   NOTE: Kohlrabi is very fibrous, so it will not reach the smoothness of purée that leafy green vegetables can.
4. Use immediately or refrigerate for 1 to 2 days.
5. For longer-term storage, transfer to freezer-safe bags. Remove as much air as possible and seal. Roasted kohlrabi will stay fresh in the freezer for between 8–12 months.
6. Remove from freezer and measure out portions for recipes as needed.

riced
1. Follow directions to remove peel and chop (steps 1–5 in prepare, above).
2. Place chopped sections in the food processor and process until riced. Uncooked kohlrabi will be processed down to firm, rice-sized pieces.
3. Use immediately or refrigerate for 1 to 2 days.
4. For longer-term storage, transfer to freezer-safe bags. Remove as much air as possible, flatten, and seal. Riced kohlrabi will stay fresh in the freezer for between 8–12 months.
5. Remove from freezer and measure out portions for recipes as needed.

---

from the Health and Wellness Coach

Nutrients Vitamin C, B6, potassium, fiber

Benefits Good for digestion, immune function, and nerve health

Fun Fact Its name comes from the German words for "cabbage" and "turnip"—and it kind of tastes like both

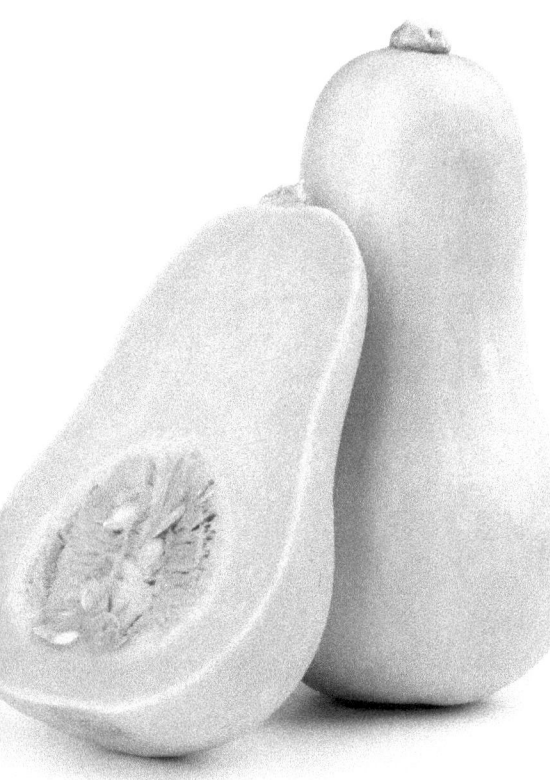

butternut squash: purée

ingredients
Whole fresh Butternut Squash

directions
1. Preheat oven to 400°F.
2. Slice the butternut squash in half lengthwise; scoop out and discard the seeds.
3. Place the halves center-side-up on the prepared baking sheet.
4. Bake for 25 to 30 minutes or until the squash can easily be pierced with a knife.
5. Remove squash from the oven; allow to cool for about 10 minutes.
6. Scoop out the flesh, place it in a food processor or blender, and blend until it achieves a smooth, creamy consistency.
7. Use immediately or refrigerate for 2 to 3 days. For longer-term storage, freeze in portions.

freezing
5. Pack into ice cube trays and freeze until solid.
6. Transfer to freezer-safe bags. Remove as much air as possible and seal.
7. Measure out individual cubes for recipes: Most ice cube trays have a 1-inch well that will hold about 1 ounce of liquid.
   8 cubes = 1 cup;
   4 cubes = ½ cup;
   2 cubes = ¼ cup
8. Properly sealed purée will stay fresh for 6 to 8 months.

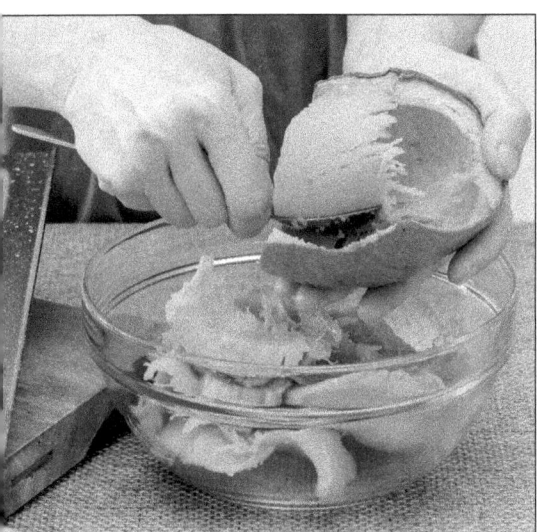

Scooping out the cooled butternut squash.

from the **Health and Wellness Coach**

Nutrients Vitamins A, C, fiber, potassium

Benefits Promotes healthy skin, immune support, and heart health

Fun Fact The seeds are edible too—roast them for a crunchy snack

carrots: riced

yield
Two medium-sized carrots (any variety) will yield approximately one cup of diced carrots.

directions
1. Use a vegetable peeler to remove the outer layer of skin.

2. Use a sharp knife to remove ½ inch from either end of the carrot and discard.

3. Rinse to remove any debris.

4. Chop the carrots into 1-inch pieces.

5. Use a food processor to dice, working in batches and pulsing until all the carrots are about rice-sized.

6. Use immediately or refrigerate for 2 to 3 days. For longer-term storage, freeze in portions.

freezing
7. Place in freezer-safe bags. Press flat to remove as much air as possible and seal. Flat packaging will make it easier to break apart after freezing to measure out and use in recipes.

8. Properly sealed carrots will stay fresh for 6 to 8 months.

from the Health and Wellness Coach

Nutrients Beta-carotene (vitamin A), fiber, potassium

Benefits Good for eyesight, skin health, and immune function

Fun Fact Cooked carrots deliver more antioxidants than raw ones

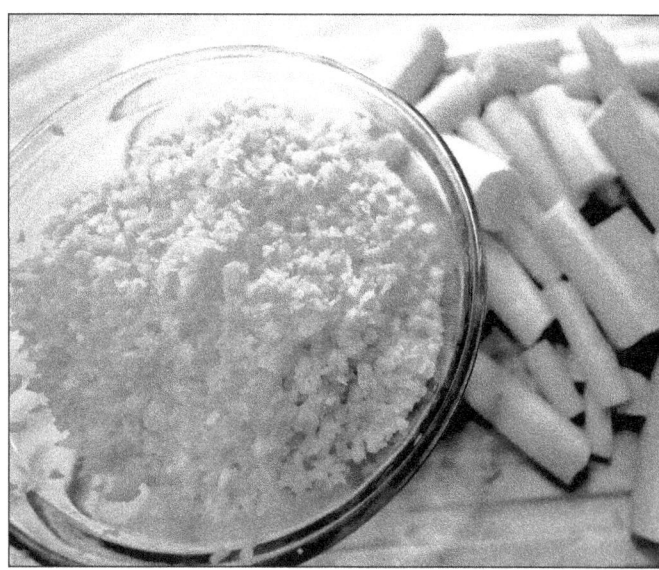

Riced carrots

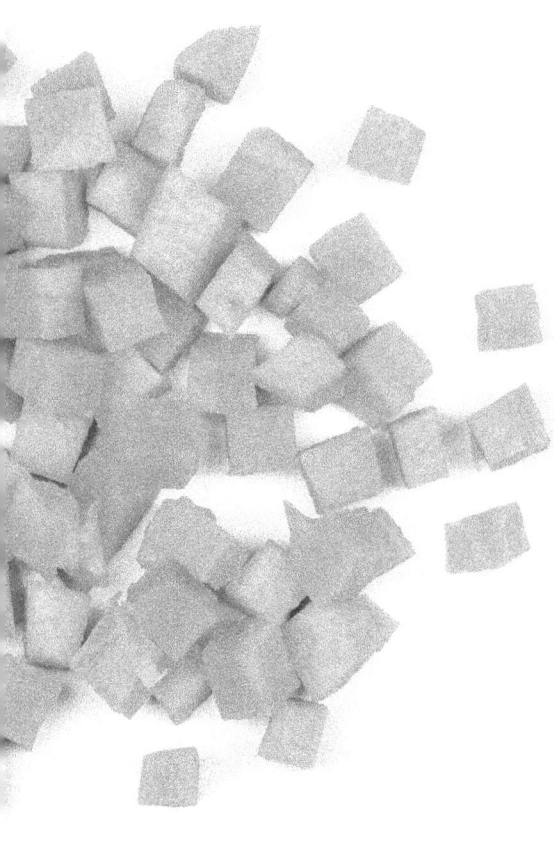

carrot juice
(without a juicer)

ingredients
2 ½ cups water

7 large carrots

yield
Ten medium-sized carrots (any variety) will yield approximately one cup of carrot juice.

directions
1. Use a vegetable peeler to remove the outer layer of skin.
2. Use a sharp knife to remove a ½ inch section from either end of the carrot and discard.
3. Rinse to remove any debris.
4. Chop into 1- or 2-inch pieces.
5. Place the chopped carrots and water in a blender or food processor.
6. Blend on high for 1 to 2 minutes until the carrots and water form a smooth mixture.
7. Strain through a colander lined with cheesecloth.
8. Save the pulp and store it separately to add to recipes like pasta sauce, soup, or stew.
9. Use immediately or refrigerate for up to 3 days.

freezing
10. Pour into ice cube trays and freeze until solid.
11. Transfer to freezer-safe bags. Remove as much air as possible and seal.
12. Measure out individual cubes for recipes: Most ice cube trays have a 1-inch well that will hold about 1 ounce of liquid.
    8 cubes = 1 cup;
    4 cubes = ½ cup;
    2 cubes = ¼ cup
13. Properly sealed, the juice will stay fresh for 6 to 8 months.

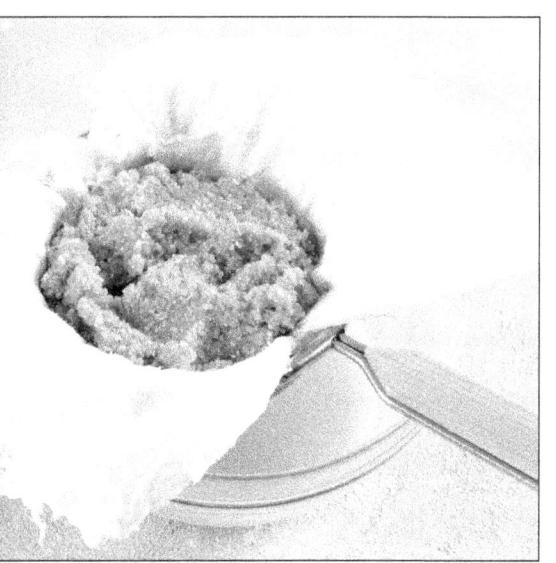

Carrots being strained through colander lined with cheesecloth.

pumpkin: purée

ingredients
Use fresh pumpkin, look for those labeled for baking or pie.

yield
One pound of pumpkin will yield approximately one and one-half cups of pumpkin purée.

directions
1. Preheat oven to 400°F.
2. Line a baking sheet with parchment paper.
3. Cut the pumpkin in half lengthwise.
4. From each half, scoop out the seeds and pulp. Place the hollowed-out pumpkin skin-side-up on the baking sheet.
5. Bake for 40 to 45 minutes until the skin can be easily pierced with a fork. Remove and place on a cooling rack.
6. Using a spoon, scoop out the cooked flesh from the skin and discard the skin.
7. Place the scooped-out flesh in a food processor and process on high until smooth.
8. Using a fine mesh sieve, strain the purée to remove larger chunks.
9. Use immediately or refrigerate for between 3 to 5 days.

freezing
1. Pack into ice cube trays and freeze until solid.
2. Transfer to freezer-safe bags. Remove as much air as possible and seal.
3. Measure out individual cubes for recipes: Most ice cube trays have a 1-inch well that will hold about 1 ounce of liquid.
   - 8 cubes = 1 cup;
   - 4 cubes = ½ cup;
   - 2 cubes = ¼ cup
4. Properly sealed purée will stay fresh for 6 to 8 months.

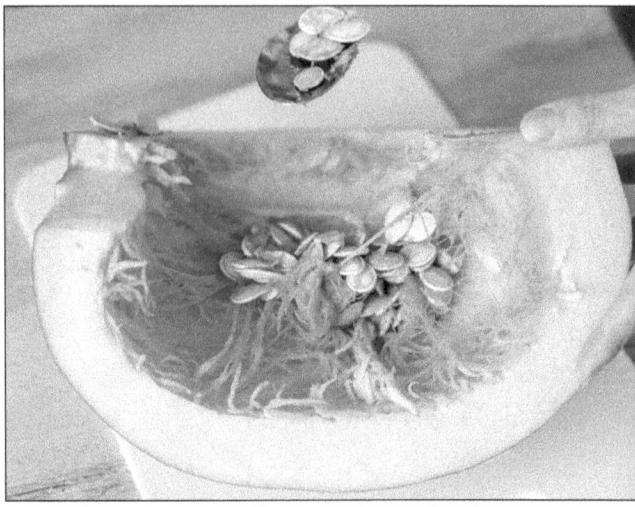

Scooping out pumpling seeds and pulp.

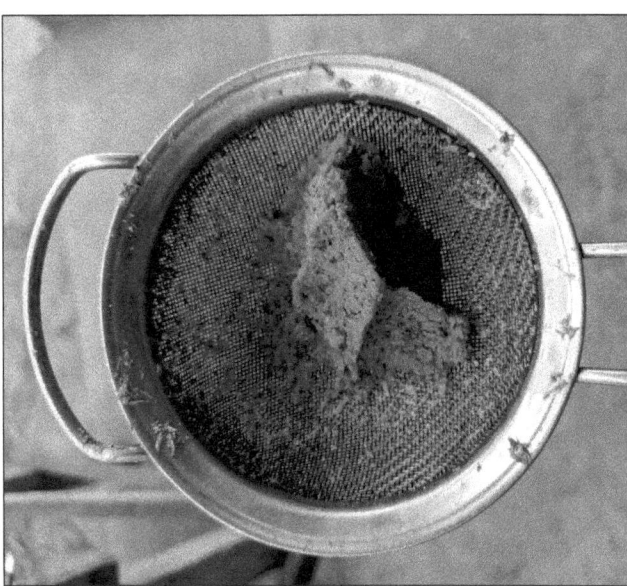

Strainging purée through fine mesh.

from the **Health and Wellness Coach**

Nutrients Beta-carotene (vitamin A), fiber, vitamin C

Benefits Eye and skin health, boosts immunity

Fun Fact Not just for pie! Pumpkin is a fruit (with seeds) and is low in calories but packed with nutrients

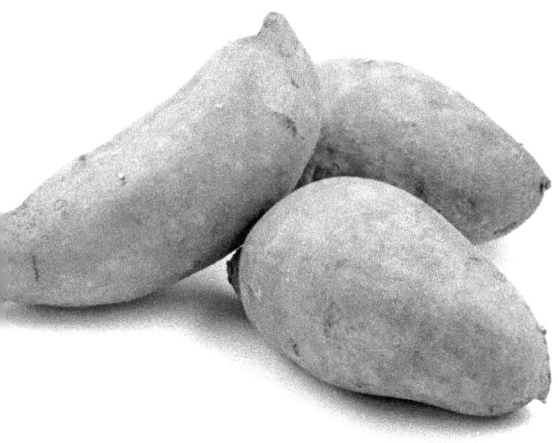

sweet potato: purée

yield
One pound of sweet potatoes (any variety) will yield approximately one and one-half cups of sweet potato purée.

directions
1. Wash to remove any dirt or debris.
2. Cook the sweet potatoes in one of three ways:
   - **Microwave Method** Pierce with a knife or fork to vent. Microwave on high for 5 to 6 minutes, or until soft.
   - **Oven Method** Preheat oven to 400°F. Pierce whole sweet potatoes with a fork and bake until tender (usually 45–60 minutes).
   - **Steam Method** Use a vegetable peeler to remove skin. Chop into 1- to 2-inch chunks. Place in a steamer basket over 2 inches of boiling water for 10 to 15 minutes, or until tender when pricked with a fork.
3. Let the potatoes cool enough to be handled.
4. For microwave and oven methods, peel away the skin and discard.
5. Chop the sweet potatoes into chunks.
6. Place in a food processor and blend at highest setting for 1 minute or until puréed and smooth.
7. Use immediately or refrigerate for 2 to 3 days. For longer-term storage, freeze in portions.

Puréed sweet potato

freezing
8. Pack into ice cube trays and freeze until solid.
9. Transfer to freezer-safe bags. Remove as much air as possible and seal.
10. Measure out individual cubes for recipes: Most ice cube trays have a 1-inch well that will hold about 1 ounce of liquid.
    - 8 cubes = 1 cup;
    - 4 cubes = ½ cup;
    - 2 cubes = ¼ cup
11. Properly sealed, purée will stay fresh for 6 to 8 months.

---

from the Health and Wellness Coach

Nutrients Beta-carotene, vitamins C and B6, potassium

Benefits Supports vision, brain health, and immune strength

Fun Fact They're technically not yams—even though the names are often used interchangeably

rutabaga (yellow turnip) riced and mashed

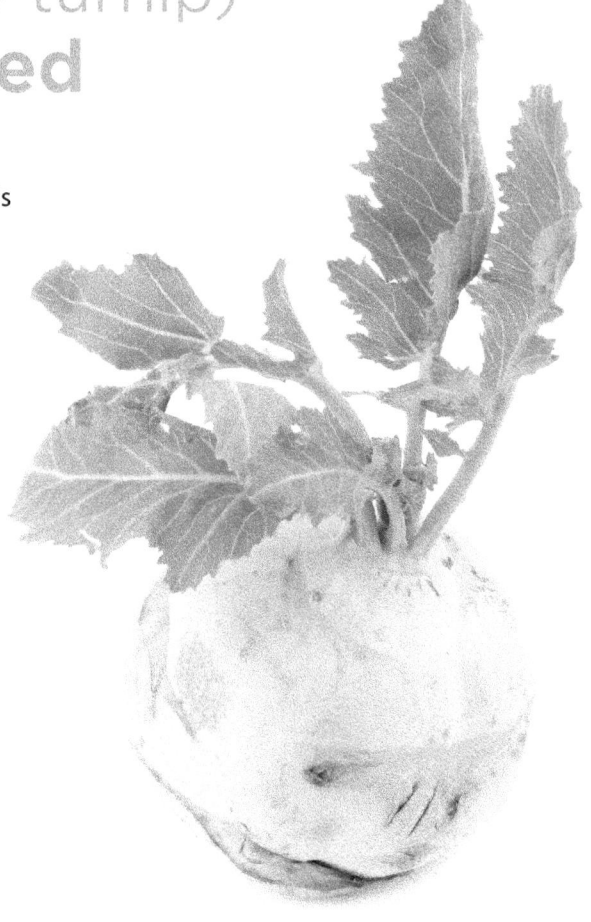

yield

One small rutabaga, about one and one-half pounds will yield approximately three cups diced.

riced

1. Rinse the rutabaga under cold running water to remove any dirt or debris.

2. Use a vegetable peeler to remove the skin and any waxy parts.

3. Chop into chunks.

4. Place in a food processor to dice, working in batches and pulsing until all the rutabaga is about rice-sized.

5. To shred, use a cheese grater or the shredder attachment on a food processor.

mashed

1. Rinse the rutabaga under cold running water to remove any dirt or debris.

2. Use a vegetable peeler to remove the skin and any waxy parts.

3. Chop into chunks.

4. Place the chopped rutabaga in a saucepan and fill with enough water to cover the chunks. Add 1 teaspoon salt.

5. Bring the pot to a boil and cook for 20 to 25 minutes or until the rutabaga is tender.

6. Drain and press with a potato masher until the mash reaches the desired consistency.

asparagus: chopped & purée

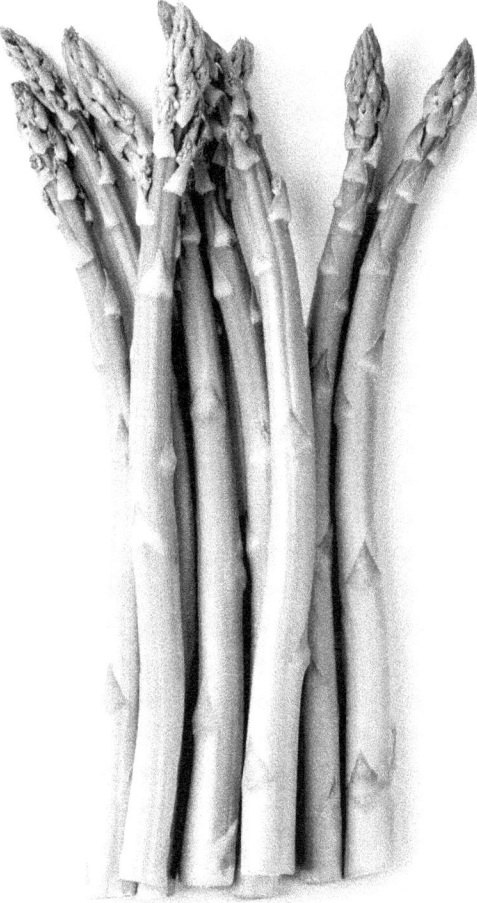

yield
Six stalks of asparagus will yield approximately one cup of diced asparagus.

chopped
1. Separate the individual spears of asparagus.
2. The base will be stiff and woody, and the spear will get more flexible as you move up. Find the spot where it starts to be flexible and snap off at that point. Discard the woody base.
3. Repeat for all the spears in the bunch.
4. Wash under cold running water.
5. Pat dry with a clean paper towel.
6. Dice by hand using a sharp knife.
7. Use immediately.

purée
8. Steam (See p. 23 for steaming options) the trimmed and cleaned asparagus for 10 minutes or until soft.
9. Place in a food processor or blender along with 2 tablespoons of the water from steaming.
10. Pulse until smooth. Freeze any asparagus that is not used immediately.

freezing
1. Pour into ice cube trays and freeze until solid.
2. Transfer to freezer-safe bags. Remove as much air as possible and seal.
3. Measure out individual cubes for recipes: Most ice cube trays have a 1-inch well that will hold about 1 ounce of liquid.
    8 cubes = 1 cup;
    4 cubes = ½ cup;
    2 cubes = ¼ cup
4. Properly sealed purée will stay fresh for up to 12 months.

---

from the Health and Wellness Coach

Nutrients Vitamins A, C, E, K, folate

Benefits Supports brain health, detoxifies the body, and promotes heart health

Fun Fact Asparagus is a natural diuretic—and it can make your pee smell funny due to a sulfur compound (totally harmless!)

broccoli: riced & minced

yield
One pound of broccoli will yield approximately two cups of minced broccoli.

directions

1. Trim off the bottom inch of the large broccoli stem and discard.

2. Using a sharp knife, cut the smaller stems to separate the florets.

3. Fill a large bowl with water. Place all the cut pieces of broccoli in the water and soak for 2 to 3 minutes. *If the broccoli is dirty, add 2 to 3 cups of white vinegar to the water before soaking.

4. Use a colander to drain. Rinse well in cold running water to remove any dirt.

5. Toss in the colander to remove excess water.

6. Cut into 1- to 2-inch pieces and place in a food processor.

7. Blend at the highest setting for 1 minute until it reaches the consistency of rice.

8. Use immediately or refrigerate in a sealed container for 2 to 3 days. For longer-term storage, freeze in portions.

freezing

9. Place in freezer-safe bags. Press flat to remove as much air as possible and seal. Flat packaging will make it easier to break the frozen chunks to measure out and use in recipes.

10. Properly sealed, broccoli will stay fresh in the freezer for 6 to 8 months.

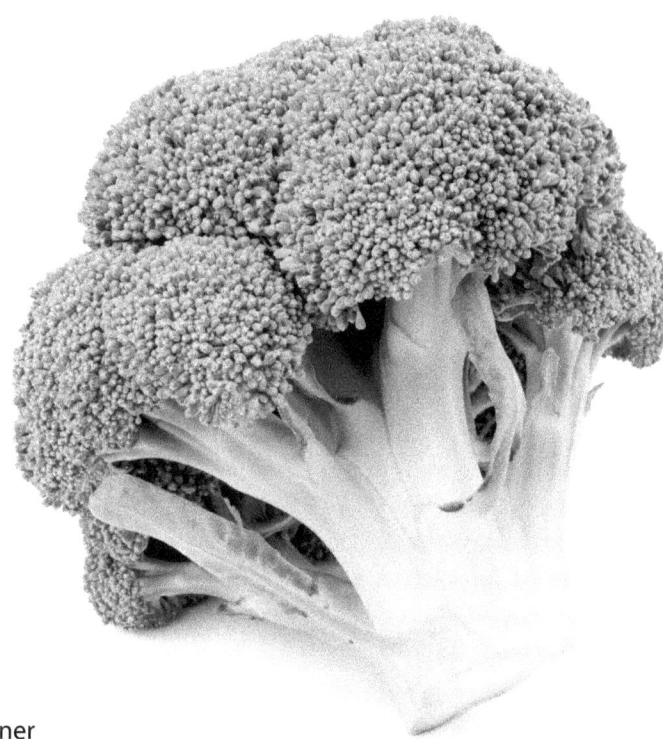

from the Health and Wellness Coach

Nutrients Vitamins C, K, A, folate, fiber

Benefits Supports bone health, immune system, and may help fight certain cancers

Fun Fact Broccoli contains more protein than most other vegetables

Brussels sprouts: minced

yield
One pound of Brussels sprouts will yield approximately two cups of minced Brussels sprouts.

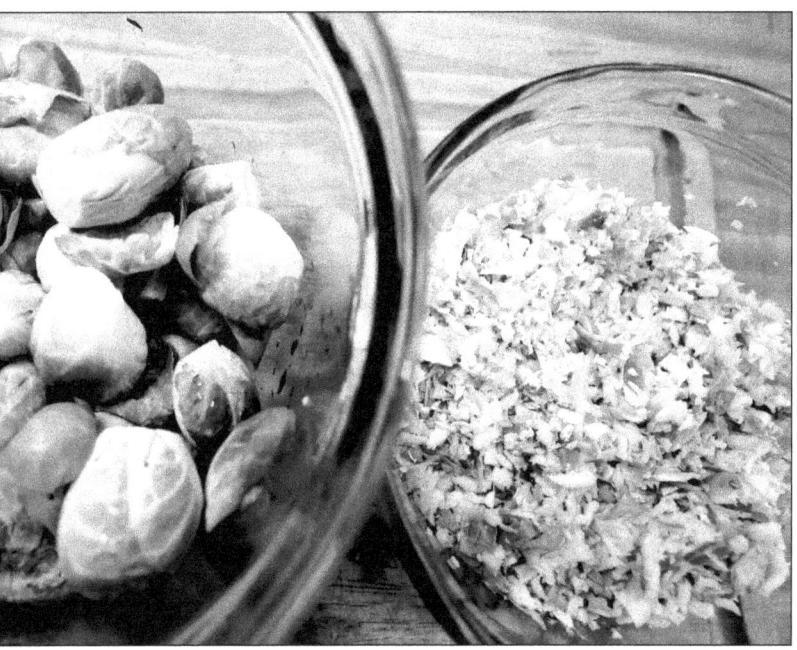

directions
1. Slice off and discard the bottom end of each Brussels sprout.
2. Remove any wilted or discolored leaves.
3. Use a food processor and pulse on high for 1 to 2 minutes until the sprouts reach the consistency of rice.
4. Use immediately or refrigerate in a sealed container for 2 to 3 days. For longer-term storage, freeze in portions.

freezing
5. Place in freezer-safe bags. Press flat to remove as much air as possible and seal. Flat packaging will make it easier to break the frozen chunks to measure out and use in recipes.
6. Properly sealed, Brussels sprouts will stay fresh in the freezer for 6 to 8 months.

---

from the **Health and Wellness Coach**

Nutrients Vitamins K, C, A, folate, fiber

Benefits Aid in detoxification, digestion, and blood clotting

Fun Fact They're mini cabbages—but way cooler. Roasting them brings out their natural sweetness

celery: minced

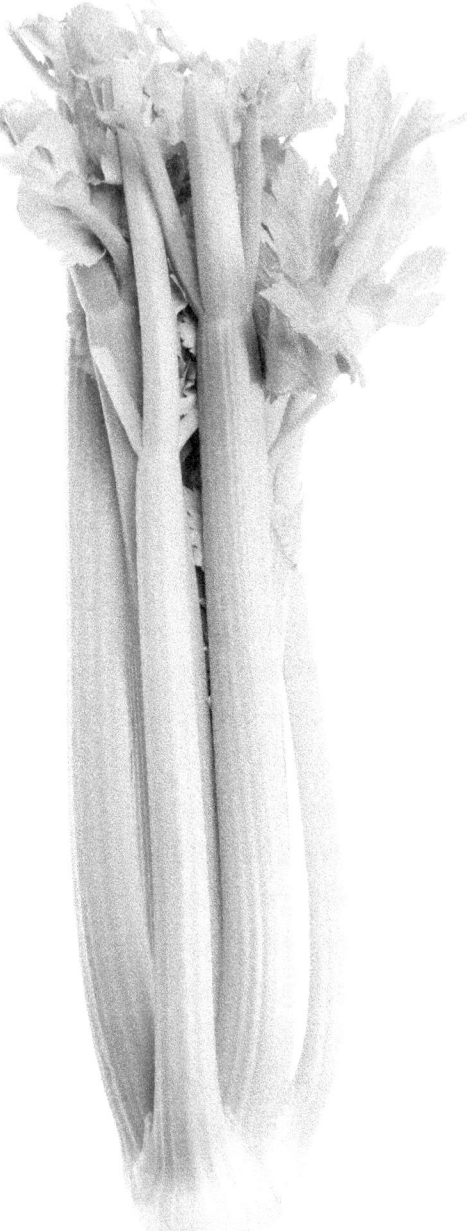

yield
Three stalks of celery will yield approximately one cup diced celery.

directions

1. Separate the individual stalks of celery by pulling them apart until they break free.

2. Cut off the tough white root at the bottom, and the leaflets at the top.

3. Rinse each rib under cold running water to remove any dirt or debris.

4. Chop the stalks into sections of about 2 inches.

5. Place in a food processor and pulse until the celery is fully minced.

6. Use immediately or refrigerate in a sealed container for 2 to 3 days. For longer-term storage, freeze in portions.

Freezing

7. Place in freezer-safe bags. Press flat to remove as much air as possible and seal. Flat packaging will make it easier to break the frozen chunks to measure out and use in recipes.

8. Properly sealed, celery will stay fresh in the freezer for 6 to 8 months.

---

from the Health and Wellness Coach

Nutrients Vitamin K, potassium, folate, fiber

Benefits Helps reduce inflammation and supports digestion

Fun Fact It's mostly water—over 95%!—but still delivers crunch and nutrients

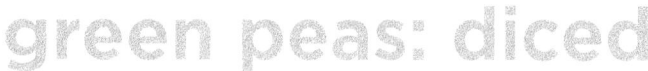
green peas: diced

yield
One pound of green peas removed from the shell will yield approximately one cup.

directions
1. Remove the green peas from their pods.
2. Rinse the shelled peas under cold running water to remove any debris.
3. Place the cleaned peas in a food processor and pulse to dice.
4. You may use a sharp knife and cutting board if you prefer, to dice the peas manually.
5. Use immediately or refrigerate in a sealed container for 2 to 3 days. For longer-term storage, freeze in portions.

freezing
6. Place in freezer-safe bags. Press flat to remove as much air as possible and seal. Flat packaging will make it easier to break the frozen chunks to measure out and use in recipes.
7. Properly sealed, green peas will stay fresh in the freezer for 6 to 8 months.

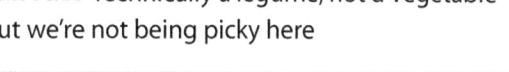

from the Health and Wellness Coach

Nutrients Protein, vitamins A, C, K, fiber

Benefits Aid in blood sugar control and digestion

Fun Fact Technically a legume, not a vegetable—but we're not being picky here

kale: purée

yield
One pound of kale (any variety), roughly five stalks around eight inches long, will yield approximately one cup of kale purée.

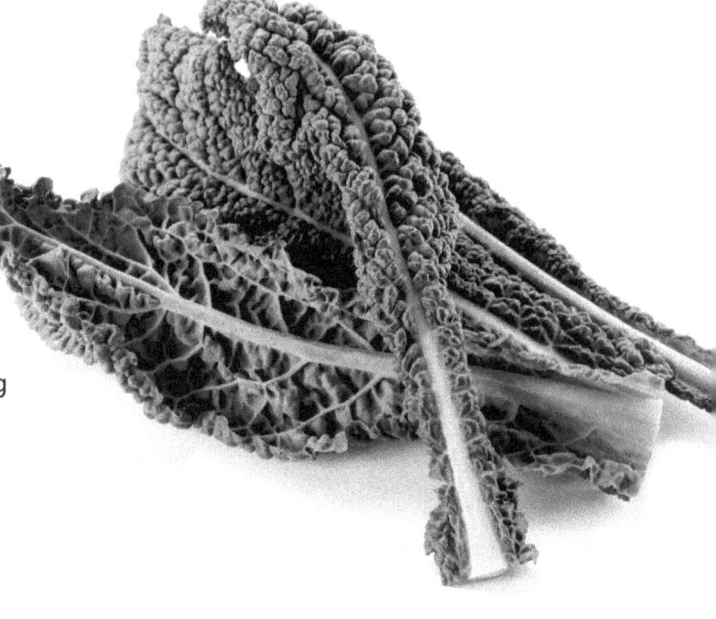

directions

1. If you have packaged kale labeled as pre-washed, remove it from the bag and give it a quick rinse under cold water.

2. For fresh kale, cut and remove stems, keeping the greens and the ribs.

3. Put the greens into a colander under cold running water to remove any dirt or debris.

4. Toss in the colander to remove excess water.

5. Cut into 1- or 2-inch pieces. Steam for 2 to 3 minutes. Place in a food processor.

6. Blend at the highest setting for 1 minute or until puréed.

7. Use immediately or refrigerate in a sealed container for 2 to 3 days. For longer-term storage, freeze in portions.

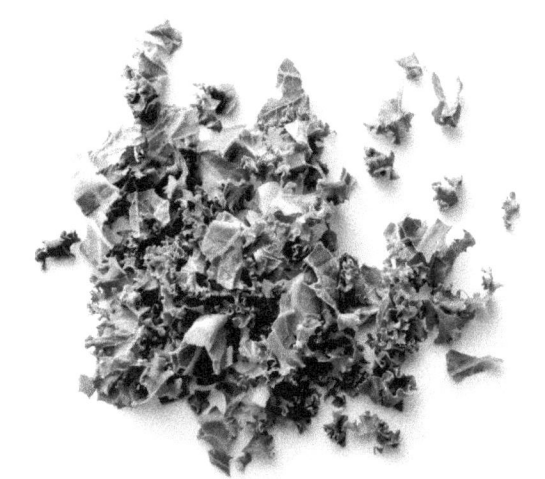

freezing

8. Pack into ice cube trays and freeze until solid.

9. Transfer to freezer-safe bags. Remove as much air as possible and seal.

10. Measure out individual cubes for recipes: Most ice cube trays have a 1-inch well that will hold about 1 ounce of liquid.
    8 cubes = 1 cup;
    4 cubes = ½ cup;
    2 cubes = ¼ cup

11. Properly sealed, the kale purée will stay fresh for 6 to 8 months.

---

from the Health and Wellness Coach

Nutrients Vitamins A, C, K, calcium, iron

Benefits Supports detox, bone strength, and heart health

Fun Fact A cup of kale has more calcium than a cup of milk

kale: juice (without a juicer)

yield
One and one-half pounds of kale (any variety), roughly seven to eight stalks around eight inches long, will yield approximately one cup of kale juice.

directions
Follow directions for **Kale Purée** from page 48:

1. If you have packaged kale labeled as pre-washed, remove it from the bag and give it a quick rinse under cold water.

2. For fresh kale, cut and remove stems, keeping the greens and the ribs.

3. Put the greens into the colander under cold running water to remove any dirt or debris.

4. Toss in a colander to remove excess water.

5. Cut into 1- or 2-inch pieces. Steam for 2 to 3 minutes. Place in a food processor.

6. Blend at the highest setting for 1 minute or until puréed.

7. Strain through a colander lined with cheesecloth.

8. Add the pulp back to the purée and store separately to add to recipes like pasta sauce, soup, or stew.

9. Use the juice immediately or refrigerate for up to 3 days.

freezing

10. Pour into ice cube trays and freeze until solid.

11. Transfer to freezer-safe bags. Remove as much air as possible and seal.

12. Measure out individual cubes for recipes: Most ice cube trays have a 1-inch well that will hold about 1 ounce of liquid.
    8 cubes = 1 cup;
    4 cubes = ½ cup;
    2 cubes = ¼ cup

13. Properly sealed, the kale juice will stay fresh for 6 to 8 months.

kale juice

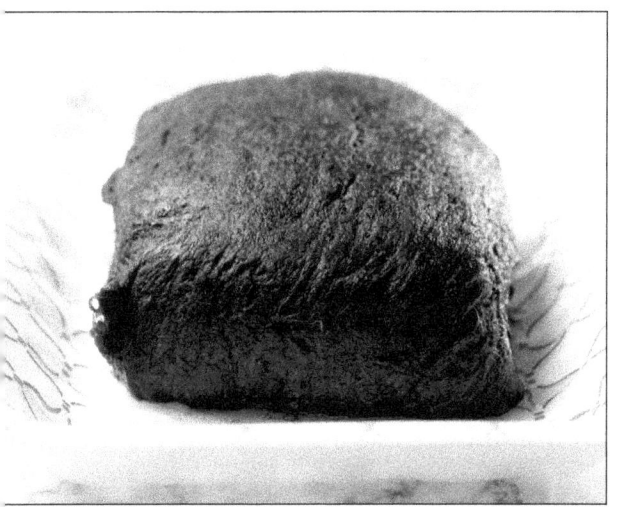

kale pulp

spinach: purée

ingredients
Fresh loose or packaged Spinach

Distilled white vinegar

yield
One pound of spinach, roughly two large bundles, will yield approximately one cup of spinach purée.

directions
1. If you have packaged spinach labeled as pre-washed, remove it from the bag and give it a quick rinse under cold water.

2. For fresh loose spinach, wash under cold running water. If spinach is mature, trim off any large stems before washing.

3. For fresh-picked spinach, put the leaves into a bowl with 8 to 10 cups of cool water and ¼ cup of 5% distilled white vinegar and keep for two minutes.

4. Rinse thoroughly and shake the spinach gently to remove excess water. It does not need to be fully dried.

5. Put into 1-or 2-inch pieces. Steam for 2 to 3 minutes. Place in a food processor.

6. Use immediately or refrigerate for 2 to 3 days. For longer-term storage, freeze in portions.

freezing
6. Pack into ice cube trays and freeze until solid.

7. Transfer to freezer-safe bags. Remove as much air as possible and seal.

9. Measure out individual cubes for recipes: Most ice cube trays have a 1-inch well that will hold about 1 ounce of liquid.
   - 8 cubes = 1 cup;
   - 4 cubes = ½ cup;
   - 2 cubes = ¼ cup

10. Properly sealed, the purée will stay fresh for 6 to 8 months.

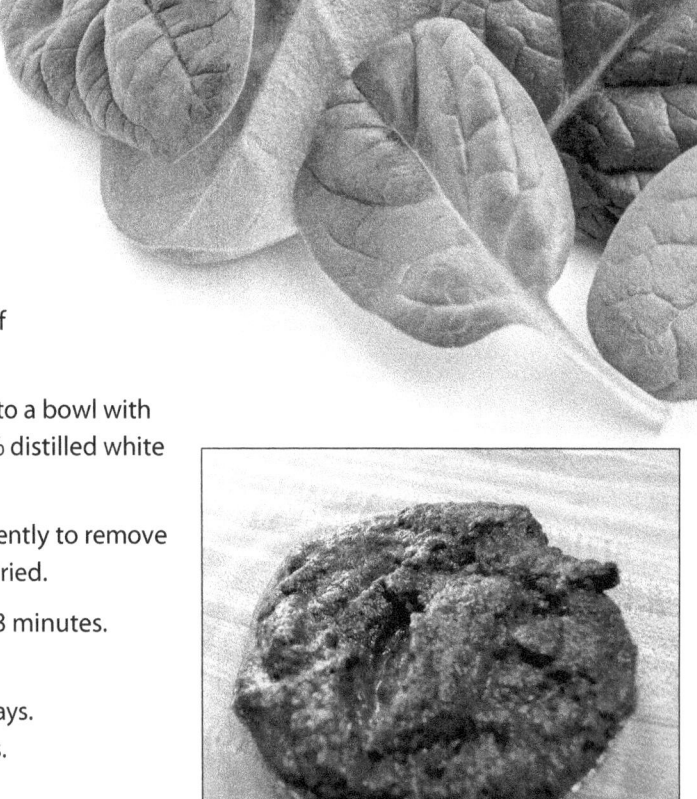

Spinach purée

---

from the Health and Wellness Coach

Nutrients Iron, magnesium, vitamin K, folate

Benefits Boosts energy, strengthens bones, and supports cell function

Fun Fact One of the best sources of plant-based iron—but pair it with vitamin C for better absorption

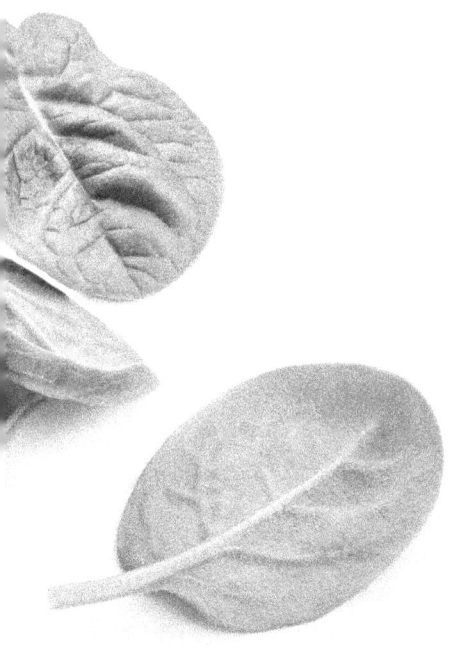

spinach juice
(without a juicer)

yield
One and one-half pound of spinach, roughly three large bundles, will yield approximately one cup of spinach juice.

directions
Follow directions for **Spinach Purée** from page 50:

1. If you have packaged spinach labeled as pre-washed, remove it from the bag and give it a quick rinse under cold water.

2. For fresh loose spinach, wash under cold running water. If spinach is mature, trim off any large stems before washing.

3. For fresh-picked spinach, put the leaves into a bowl with 8 to 10 cups of cool water and ¼ cup of 5% distilled white vinegar and keep for two minutes.

4. Rinse thoroughly and shake the spinach gently to remove excess water. It does not need to be fully dried.

5. Put into 1-o r2-inch pieces. Steam for 2 to 3 minutes. Place in a food processor.

6. Strain through a colander lined with cheesecloth.

7. Add pulp back to the purée and store separately to add to recipes like pasta sauce, soup, or stew.

8. Use juice immediately or refrigerate for up to 3 days.

freezing
9. Pour into ice cube trays and freeze until solid.

10. Transfer to freezer-safe bags. Remove as much air as possible and seal.

11. Measure out individual cubes for recipes: Most ice cube trays have a 1-inch well that will hold about 1 ounce of liquid.
    - 8 cubes = 1 cup;
    - 4 cubes = ½ cup;
    - 2 cubes = ¼ cup

12. Properly sealed, the juice will stay fresh for 6 to 8 months.

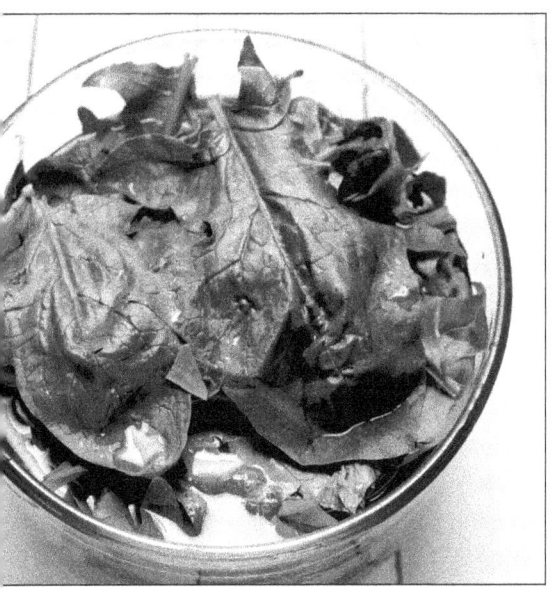

Spinach in bowl of water and distilled white vinegar

Swiss chard: purée

yield
One pound of Swiss chard, roughly two large bunches about ten stalks each, will yield approximately one cup of Swiss chard purée.

directions
1. If you have packaged Swiss chard labeled as pre-washed, remove it from the bag and rinse under cold water.

2. For fresh loose Swiss chard, wash thoroughly in a colander under cold running water. If mature, trim off any large stems before washing.

3. For fresh-picked chard, put the leaves into a bowl with 8 to 10 cups of cool water and ¼ cup of 5% distilled white vinegar and keep for two minutes.

4. Rinse thoroughly and shake gently to remove excess water. The leaves do not need to be fully dried.

5. Place in a food processor and blend at the highest setting for 1 minute or until puréed.

6. Use immediately or refrigerate for 2 to 3 days. For longer-term storage, freeze in portions.

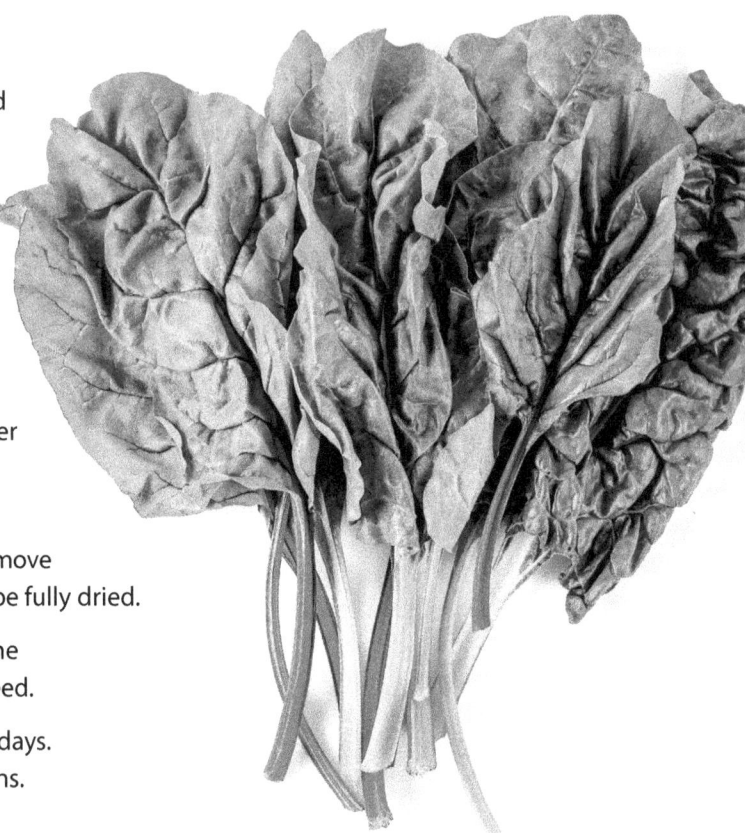

freezing
7. Pack into ice cube trays and freeze until solid.

8. Transfer to freezer-safe bags. Remove as much air as possible and seal.

9. Measure out individual cubes for recipes: Most ice cube trays have a 1-inch well that will hold about 1 ounce of liquid.
    8 cubes = 1 cup;
    4 cubes = ½ cup;
    2 cubes = ¼ cup

10. Properly sealed, the purée will stay fresh for 6 to 8 months.

---

from the **Health and Wellness Coach**

Nutrients Vitamins K, A, C, magnesium, iron

Benefits Supports blood sugar regulation and bone health

Fun Fact The vibrant stems are edible and packed with nutrients—don't toss them!

zucchini: shredded

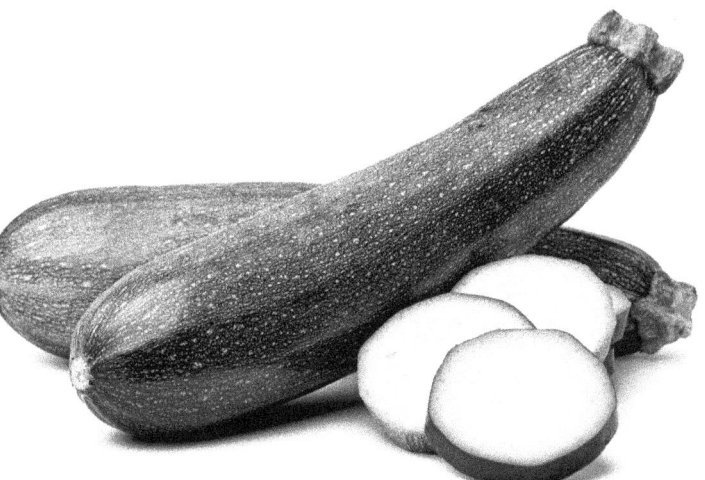

yield
One pound of zucchini will yield approximately three cups shredded when excess water is removed.

directions
1. Wash zucchini under cool running water.
2. If needed, use a vegetable brush to remove any dirt or debris.
3. Pat dry with a paper towel.
4. On a cutting board, trim away the stem and root end of the zucchini.
5. Rough chop into 2- to 3-inch pieces.
6. Use a food processor with the fine shredding disc attachment, feeding pieces through the machine to shred.
7. Place in a medium-sized bowl and allow to set for 3 to 5 minutes, then drain excess liquid through a colander.
8. Store covered in a refrigerator for 2 to 3 days.

TIP: Save the strained zucchini water to use in smoothies, add lemon for a refreshing drink, or add in place of water in any recipe. See page 54 for more tips. It's rich in folic acid, vitamins C & K, manganese, and antioxidants to keep you hydrated and energized!

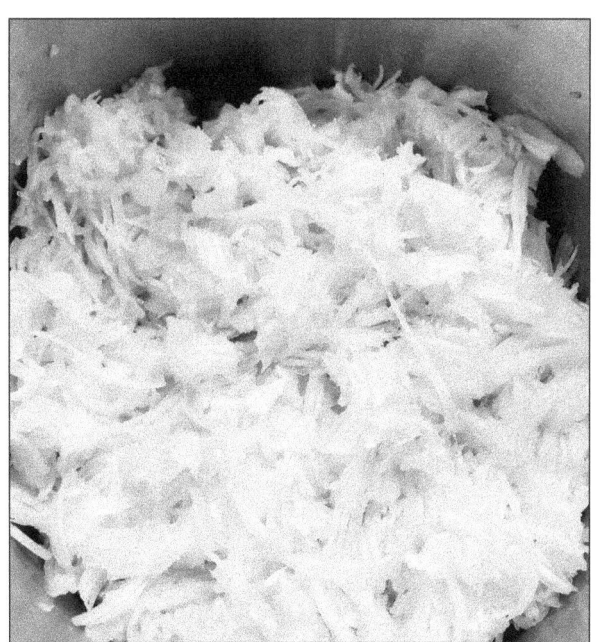

shredded zucchini

---

from the Health and Wellness Coach

Nutrients Vitamin C, manganese, fiber

Benefits Aids digestion, reduces inflammation, and supports hydration

Fun Fact Zucchini flowers are edible—and a delicacy in many cultures

Uses for Cauliflower and Zucchini Water (Juice)

Smoothies Add to your favorite smoothie recipe.

Infused Water Include with fruit in your infused water.

Cocktails + Mocktails Veggie juice can give a great flavor kick to cocktails (and mocktails).

Add to Tea Add a spoonful to hot tea to get a flavor boost as well as a nutritional boost!

Instant Mixes When the instructions read, "Add water" use an eqaul amount of veggie juice.

Rice + Quinoa When making instant rice or quinoa, measure out an equal amount of veggie juice to use in place of water for cooking.

Soup Use veggie juice instead of adding broth to a soup recipe for a flavor and nutritional boost.

Oatmeal Use veggie juice instead of water to give instant oatmeal a flavor and nutritional boost.

Ice Cubes Pour veggie juice into ice cube trays and freeze. Add to water, juice, cocktails, or mocktails for nutrition and flavor.

Gravy Use veggie juice instead of water when making gravies.

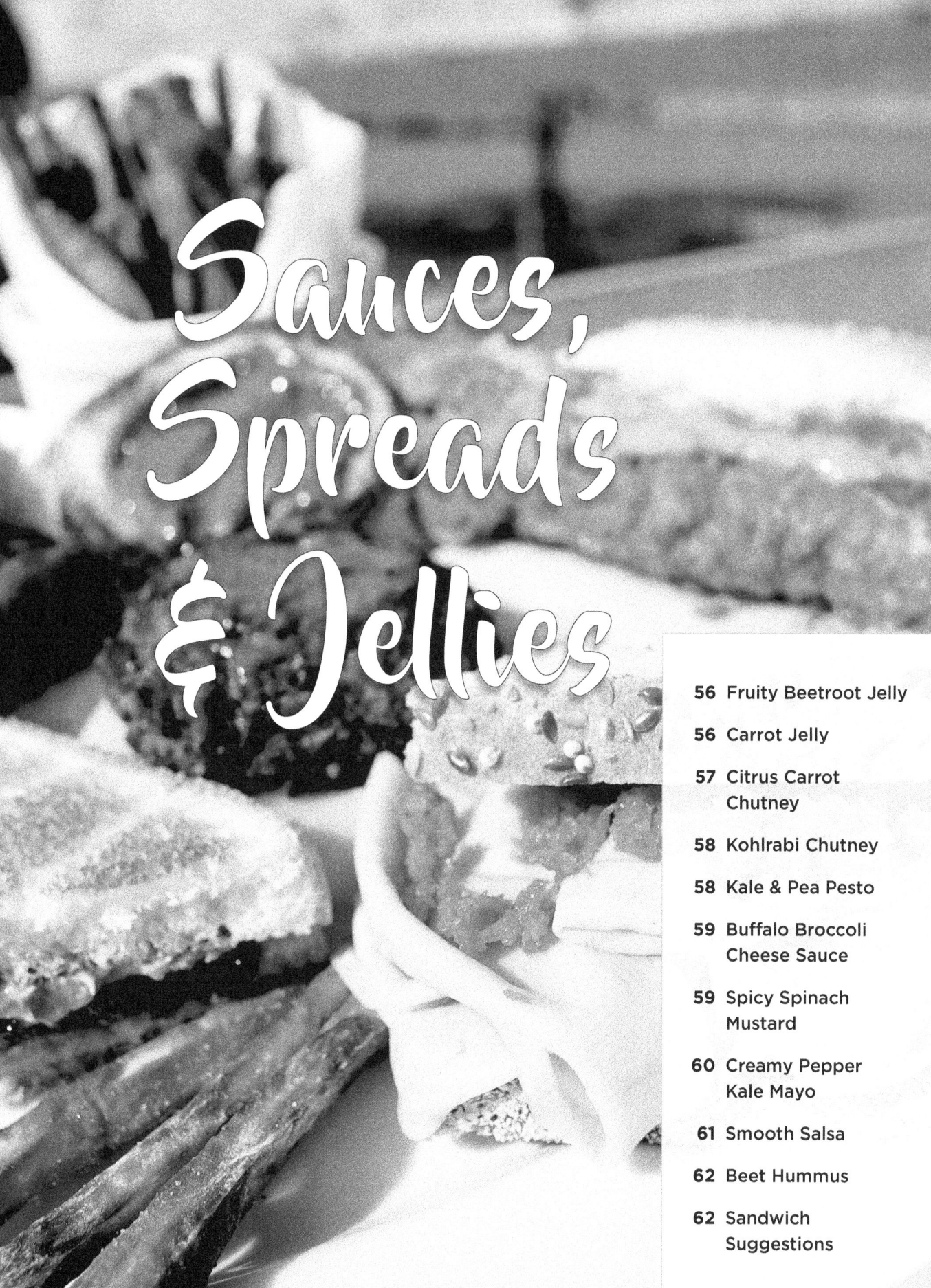

Sauces, Spreads & Jellies

- **56** Fruity Beetroot Jelly
- **56** Carrot Jelly
- **57** Citrus Carrot Chutney
- **58** Kohlrabi Chutney
- **58** Kale & Pea Pesto
- **59** Buffalo Broccoli Cheese Sauce
- **59** Spicy Spinach Mustard
- **60** Creamy Pepper Kale Mayo
- **61** Smooth Salsa
- **62** Beet Hummus
- **62** Sandwich Suggestions

Fruity Beetroot Jelly

ingredients

- 2 cups **beet juice** (strained from purée)
- 1 cup unsweetened fruit juice (plum, grape, etc) or use 1 cup fresh strawberries
- 2 tablespoons lemon juice
- 1 package Sure-Jell fruit pectin
- 3 cups sugar

directions

1. In a large stockpot over high heat, bring **beet juice,** fruit juice, and lemon juice to a boil.
2. Stir in the pectin.
3. Add the sugar and return to a boil, allowing the mixture to boil for one minute.
4. Spoon the jelly into clean, sterile, half-pint (8 ounce) or pint (1-cup) canning jars leaving ¼-inch head space. Affix the lids and rings.
5. Store in a refrigerator or water bath for longer storage.

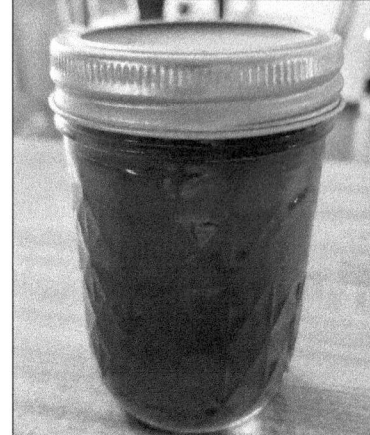

Carrot Jelly

ingredients

- 2 cups carrot juice
- 2 ⅓ cups granulated sugar
- 1 package Sure-Jell fruit pectin
- 2 tablespoons brandy
- 1 tablespoon lemon zest
- ⅓ cup lemon juice

directions

1. In a large stockpot over high heat, stir carrot juice and sugar until the sugar dissolves. Continue stirring until the mixture begins to boil.
2. Add Sure-Jell and return to a boil.
3. Boil for 5 minutes, stirring constantly.
4. Remove from heat.
5. Stir in brandy, lemon zest, and lemon juice.
6. Spoon the jelly into clean, sterile, half-pint (8oz) or pint (1-cup) canning jars leaving ¼-inch head space. Affix the lids and rings.
7. Store in a refrigerator for up to 3 weeks or water bath for longer storage.

Citrus Carrot Chutney

directions

1. Use a vegetable peeler to remove the outer layer of the skin.
2. Use a sharp knife to remove half an inch from either end of the carrot and discard.
3. Rinse to remove any debris. Chop into 2- to 3-inch pieces, then use a food processor to mince.
4. Zest and juice the lemon and the oranges. Discard the peels.
5. In a large stockpot over high heat, stir together the juice and zest from the oranges and lemons. Add the diced carrots.
6. Cook over medium heat for 8 to 10 minutes.
7. Add the sugars and spices. Stir until the sugar has completely dissolved.
8. Bring to a boil.
9. Boil for 3 minutes while stirring constantly.
10. Remove from heat and stir in the walnuts.
11. Spoon the chutney into clean, sterile, half-pint (8-ounce) or pint (1-cup) canning jars, leaving ¼-inch head space. Affix the lids and rings.
12. Store in a refrigerator for up to 3 weeks or water bath for longer storage.

TIP: Use as a relish, add cream cheese and serve with crackers, or use to top grilled chicken or pork chops.

ingredients

10 medium carrots

2 oranges

1 lemon

1½ cup granulated sugar

¾ cup dark brown sugar

½ tsp allspice

½ tsp ground ginger

½ tsp ground cinnamon

½ tsp vanilla extract

½ cup walnuts, chopped

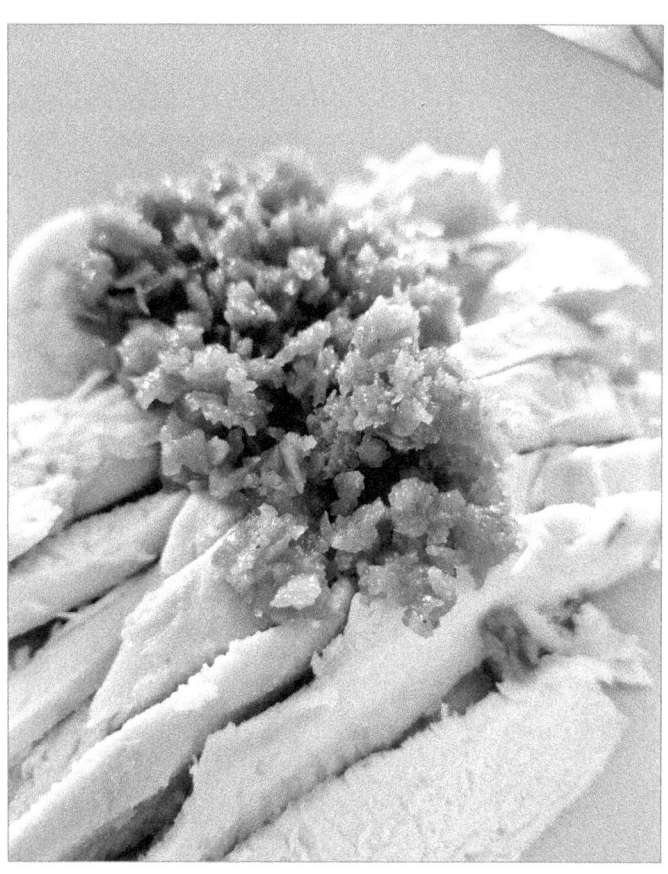

Sauces, Spreads & Jellies

Kohlrabi Chutney

ingredients

- ¼ cup vegetable oil
- 1 tablespoon coriander seed
- 1 tablespoon cumin seed
- 1 teaspoon ground cinnamon
- 2 tablespoons ginger
- 1 cup apple cider vinegar
- 1 cup raisins
- 1 cup diced apples
- ½ cup dried cranberry
- 1 teaspoon salt
- 1½ cups finely **minced kohlrabi**
- 1 cup riced carrots
- ¼ cup diced onion

directions

1. In a large stockpot over medium heat, blend the vegetable oil, coriander seed, cumin seed, cinnamon, and ginger.
2. Stir continuously and cook for 3 to 5 minutes until well-mixed and the oil has turned a warm brown color.
3. Add apple cider vinegar, apples, dried cranberries, raisins, and salt, and bring to a simmer while stirring constantly.
4. Simmer (lightly bubbling) for 3 to 4 minutes until the mixture begins to thicken.
5. Add the **kohlrabi,** carrot, and onions; stir to coat completely.
6. Bring to a boil.
7. Boil for one minute.
8. Remove from heat and cool.
9. Store in sealed containers in a refrigerator for at least 24 hours before serving.

Kale & Pea Pesto

ingredients

- ½ cup chopped peas
- 1 cup **kale purée**
- ¼ cup chopped cashews or pine nuts
- ½ grated Parmesan cheese
- 1 tablespoon lemon juice
- ½ teaspoon salt
- ¼ teaspoon pepper
- ½ teaspoon red pepper flakes
- 3 tablespoons olive oil

directions

1. Using a food processor, pulse the chopped peas and **kale purée,** blending until it forms a smooth paste.
2. Add the nuts, Parmesan cheese, lemon juice, salt, pepper, and red pepper flakes to the food processor and pulse to combine completely.
3. Transfer the mixture to a medium bowl. Slowly add olive oil and blend with a whisk until the ingredients are thoroughly mixed and the texture is creamy.

Buffalo Broccoli Cheese Sauce

directions

1. In a medium microwave-safe bowl, combine and mix all the ingredients.
2. Microwave for 1 minute. Stir to blend.
3. Use this sauce as a dip or sandwich spread.
4. Store any unused portion in a sealed container in the refrigerator.

ingredients

One 15-ounce can of nacho cheese sauce

¼ cup buffalo wing sauce

½ cup riced broccoli

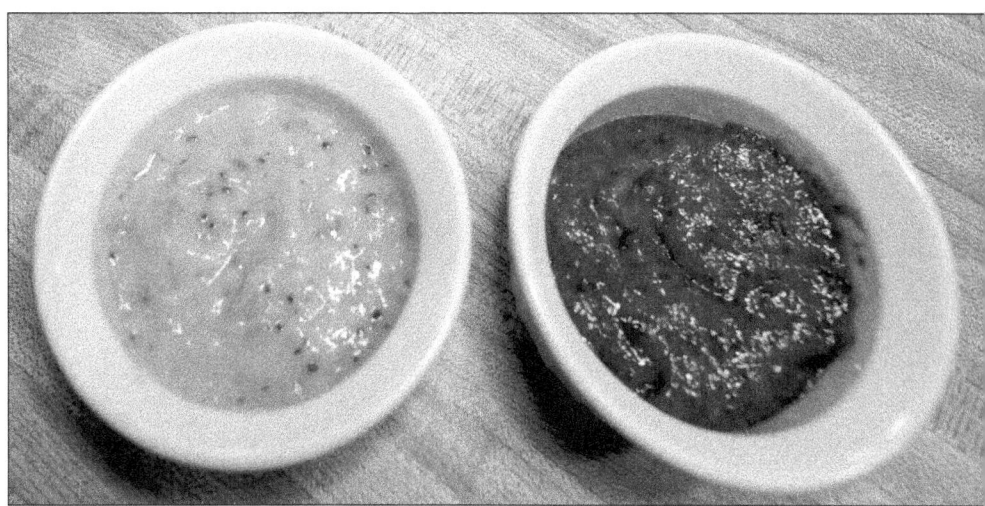

Buffalo Broccoli Cheese Sauce (left)

Spicy Spinach Mustard (right)

Spicy Spinach Mustard

directions

1. In a medium bowl, mix the dry mustard and vinegar. Whisk to blend. Cover and let the mixture stand at room temperature for 8 to 12 hours.
2. In a small saucepan, whisk egg yolk and sugar to blend. Slowly add the prepared mustard–vinegar mixture, habanero powder, and **puréed spinach**. Simmer over low heat until thickened.
3. Remove from heat and cool.

ingredients

⅓ to ½ cup dry mustard

½ cup white vinegar

1 egg yolk

½ cup sugar

½ teaspoon ground habanero powder

¼ cup **puréed spinach**

Creamy Pepper Kale Mayo

ingredients

- 2 cups fresh kale, packed into measuring cups
- 2 cloves garlic, finely diced
- 1 egg at room temperature
- 1 tablespoon apple cider vinegar
- 1 tablespoon Dijon mustard
- ¾ teaspoon salt
- 1 cup canola oil
- 1 teaspoon fresh-ground pepper
- 4 tablespoons lemon juice
- 1 teaspoon lemon zest

directions

1. Clean the kale and remove the stems. Place the kale in a food processor and pulse until puréed. Add the diced garlic and blend.

2. Scrape into a bowl and set aside.

3. Place the egg in the food processor and blend for 20 to 30 seconds. Add Dijon mustard, apple cider vinegar, and salt. Blend for an additional 20 to 30 seconds.

4. Use a scraper to clean the sides of the bowl, then, taking 2 to 3 minutes, slowly add the oil ⅛ cup at a time to allow the ingredients to blend and thicken.

5. Mix in the kale and garlic purée and blend.

6. Add fresh ground pepper, lemon juice, and lemon zest.

7. Store covered in the refrigerator for up to a week.

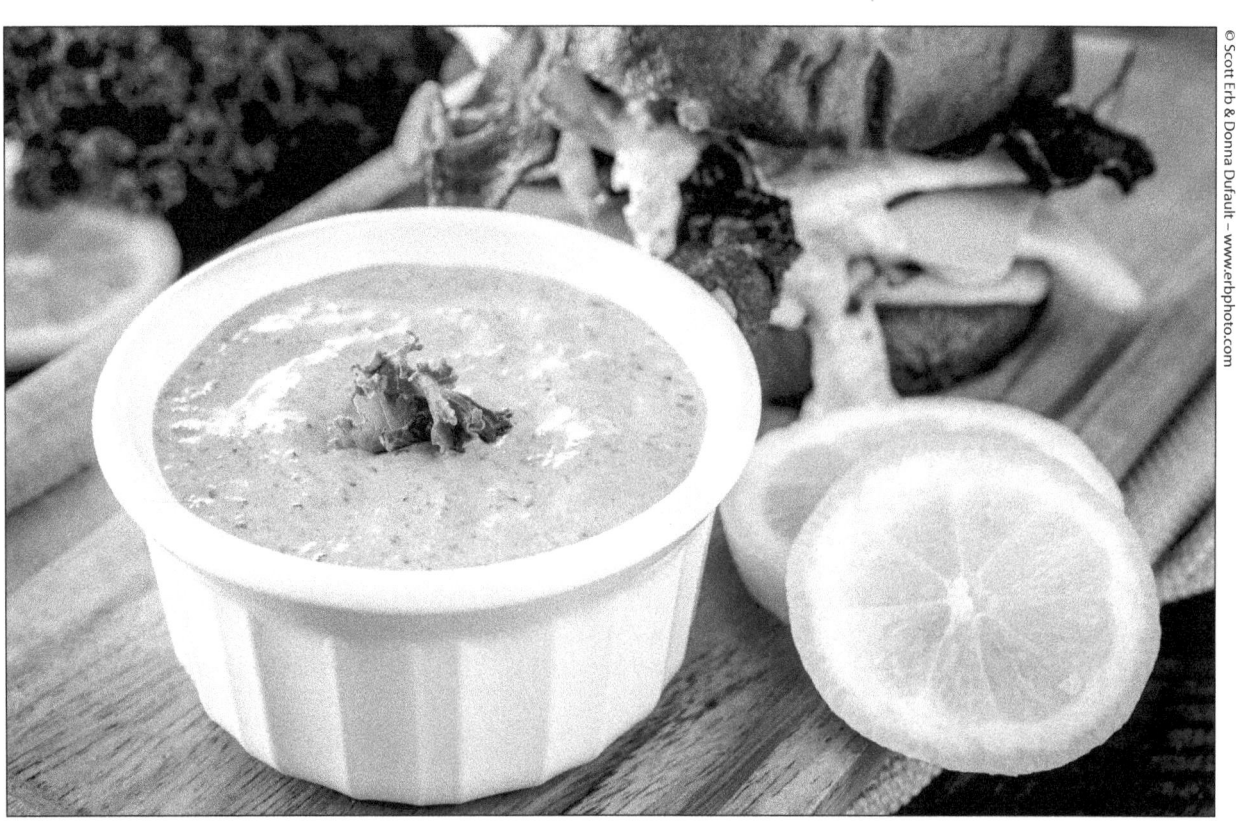

Smooth Salsa

directions

1. Combine all the ingredients in a large stockpot over medium heat.
2. Bring to a boil.
3. Boil for 2 minutes.
4. Reduce heat to a simmer and cook uncovered for 30 to 45 minutes or until thickened.
5. Store in sealed containers in the refrigerator or freeze in airtight bags for up to 8 months.

ingredients

8 cups **puréed tomato**

1 cup **puréed red bell pepper**

2 diced leeks

2 jalapeño peppers, seeded and puréed

¾ cup tomato paste

⅔ cup condensed tomato soup

½ cup white vinegar

2 tablespoons sugar

1 tablespoon salt

2 tablespoons onion powder

4½ teaspoons garlic powder

1 tablespoon cayenne pepper

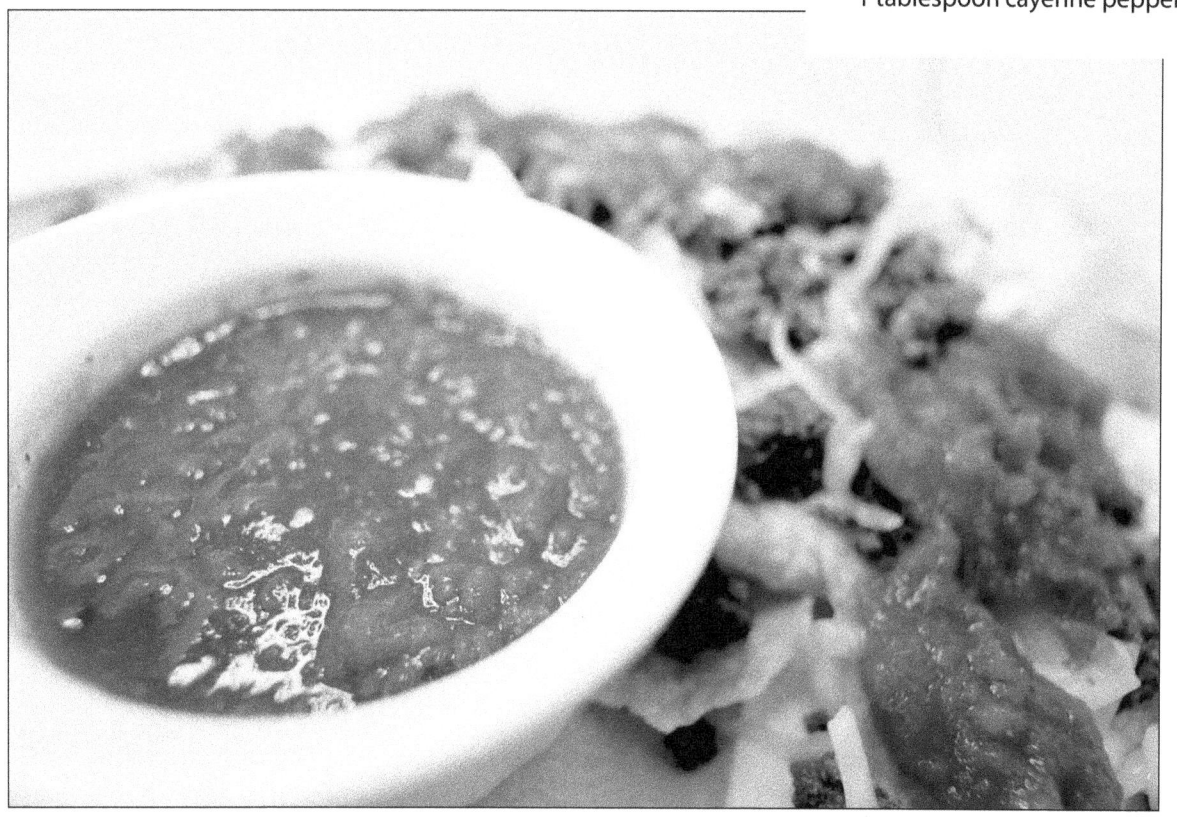

Sauces, Spreads & Jellies

Beet Hummus

ingredients

- 1½ cups **puréed beets**
- 1 tablespoon orange juice
- 4 tablespoons lemon juice
- zest of 1 large lemon (about 1 tablespoon)
- Two 15-oz cans of cooked chickpeas, drained
- 2 large garlic cloves, minced
- ¼ teaspoon salt
- ¼ teaspoon pepper
- ¼ cup extra virgin olive oil

directions

1. In a blender or food processor, combine **puréed beets,** orange juice, lemon juice, and lemon zest. Pulse until smooth.
2. Add chickpeas, garlic, salt and pepper, and pulse until smooth.
3. Place in a large bowl and mix in olive oil.
4. Store in an airtight container in the refrigerator for up to 4 to 5 days.

IDEAS: Serve as a dip with pita chips or crackers, add as a sandwich spread, or substitute for mayonnaise in recipes.

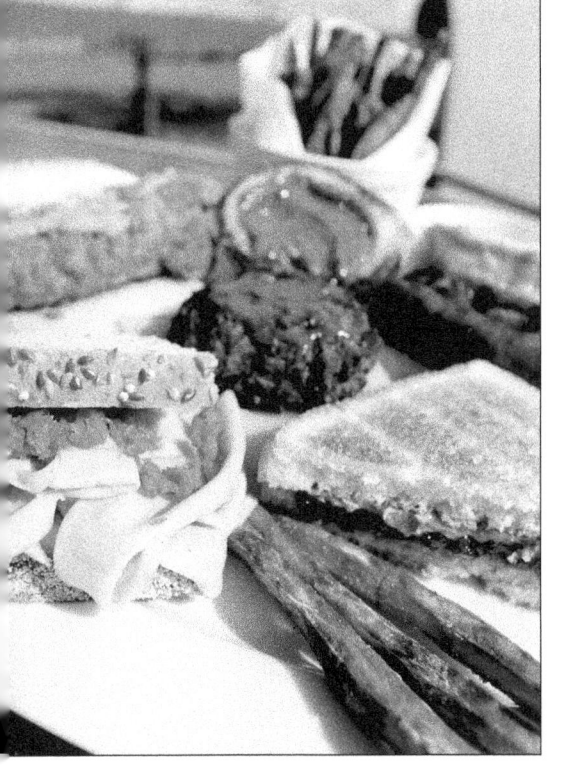

Sandwich Suggestions

Recipes for sauces/spreads at the beginning of the section, then sandwich assembly.

Smoked Turkey with Beet Hummus and Swiss on sourdough bread

Ham with Spicy Spinach Mustard and pepperjack on a multigrain roll

Fried Fish with Citrus Carrot Chutney in Pita Bread

Roast Beef with Buffalo Broccoli Cheese Sauce on a pretzel bun

Gourmet Grilled Cheese: Buffalo broccoli cheese sauce with Swiss and cheddar cheese on Texas Toast. If you like tangy, add horseradish!

PBBJ: Peanut Butter & Fruity Beetroot Jelly on potato bread

Spicy Meatball Provolone on Spinach Roll

Chicken Mozzarella with Creamy Pepper Kale on Brioche Bun

Sauces, Spreads & Jellies

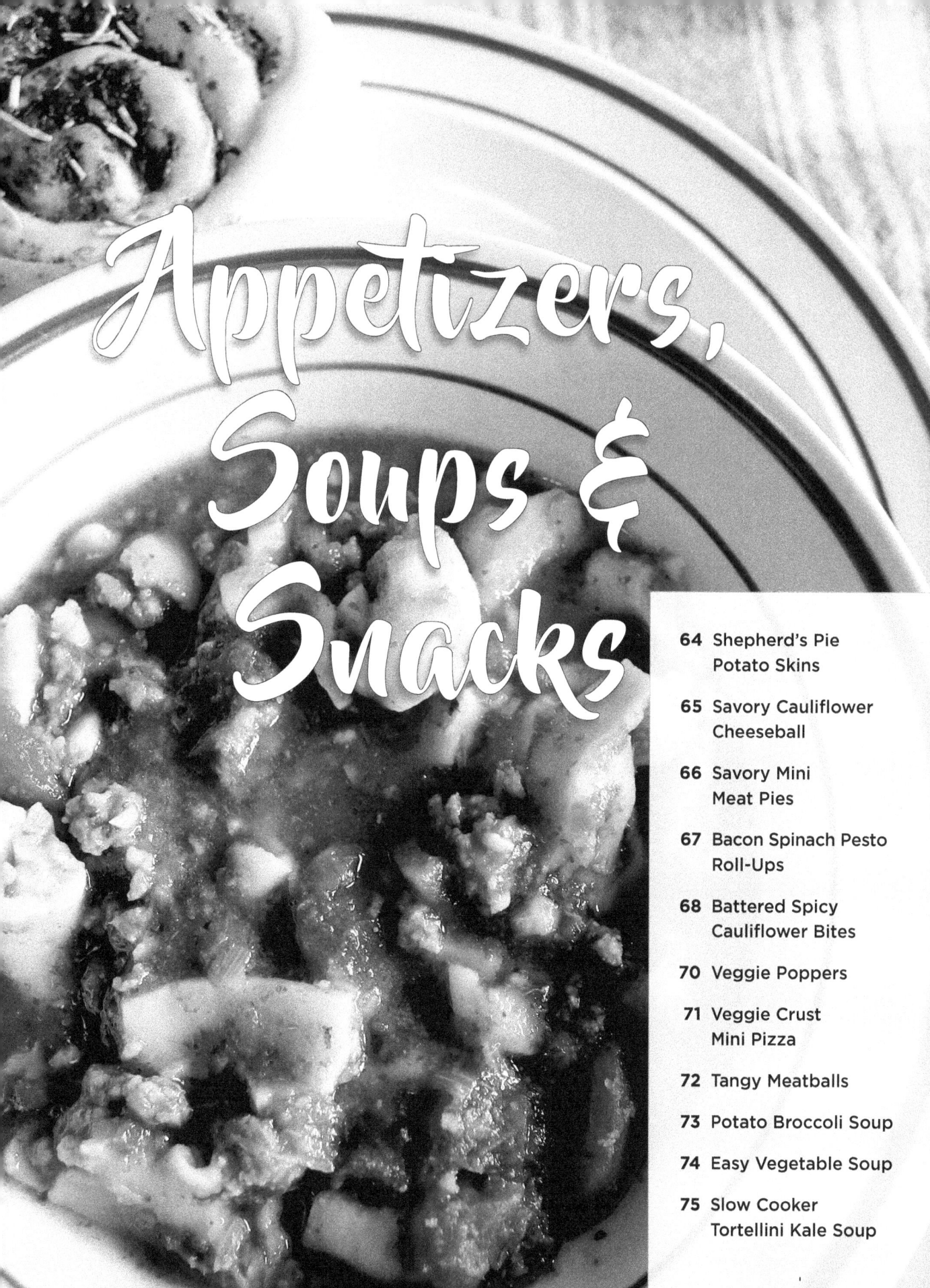

Appetizers, Soups & Snacks

- **64** Shepherd's Pie Potato Skins
- **65** Savory Cauliflower Cheeseball
- **66** Savory Mini Meat Pies
- **67** Bacon Spinach Pesto Roll-Ups
- **68** Battered Spicy Cauliflower Bites
- **70** Veggie Poppers
- **71** Veggie Crust Mini Pizza
- **72** Tangy Meatballs
- **73** Potato Broccoli Soup
- **74** Easy Vegetable Soup
- **75** Slow Cooker Tortellini Kale Soup

Shepherd's Pie Potato Skins

ingredients

4 large potatoes, washed and patted dry

½ to 1 cup milk

2 tablespoons of butter

½ teaspoon salt

¼ teaspoon pepper

1 tablespoon olive oil

1 tablespoon butter

½ cup minced leeks

2 cloves of garlic

1 pound ground beef

1 cup riced carrots

½ cup minced green peas

½ cup whole kernel corn

2 tablespoons flour

1 cup beef bouillon

½ cup water

½ teaspoon salt

1 tablespoon granulated garlic

½ teaspoon dried thyme

½ teaspoon dried oregano

Black pepper

Shredded cheddar cheese (optional)

directions

1. Preheat oven to 400°F.

2. Bake potatoes for 60 to 75 minutes (*Working day tip:* Cook these in the crockpot! Prick the potatoes with a fork several times, then rub with olive oil and season with salt before wrapping them in foil, and place in the crockpot over a low flame for 6 to 7 hours).

3. When the potatoes are fully cooked, cool enough to handle.

4. Laying each potato lengthwise, slice about ⅔ of the top skin to expose the white flesh.

5. Scoop out the flesh, leaving about ¼-inch to ½-inch along the edges so that the hollowed-out potato retains its shape. Place the removed flesh in a large bowl and continue until all the potatoes are hollowed out.

6. Arrange the hollowed-out potatoes on a baking sheet and set aside.

7. Add milk, butter, salt, and pepper to the potato flesh kept in the bowl. For smooth potatoes, use an electric hand mixer on low. For a chunkier mix, hand mash with a potato masher until you achieve the desired consistency. Set aside.

8. In a large skillet over medium heat, melt the butter with the olive oil. Add diced fresh garlic and minced leeks. Sauté for about 2 minutes until softened.

9. Add the ground beef and cook for 7 to 10 minutes until fully browned.

10. Add flour and spices, stirring to blend with the cooked ground beef.

11. Add the beef bouillon, water, carrots, peas, and corn.

12. Simmer and allow to cook down until thickened. Turn off the burner and cool.

13. Preheat oven to 350°F.

Shepherd's Pie Potato Skins (continued)

14. *To assemble the potatoes:* Fill each hollowed-out potato skin with the ground beef mixture up to just below the top. Use a spoon to top the ground beef with mashed potatoes. For a more formal look, use a piping bag with a large star nozzle. Add the mashed potatoes to the bag and pipe onto the filled potato skins.

15. Add cheddar cheese if desired.

16. Bake for 15 to 20 minutes until the stuffed potatoes are slightly brown on top.

Savory Cauliflower Cheeseball

directions

1. In a large bowl, blend cream cheese, cauliflower rice, onion powder, garlic, ginger, and Worcestershire sauce until smooth.

2. Add the cheeses and stir until thoroughly mixed.

3. Using your hands, shape the mix into a ball.

4. Spread everything bagel seasoning on a plate and roll the cheeseball over it until the ball is covered fully in the spice.

5. Wrap the cheeseball in plastic and chill until firm.

6. Serve with crackers.

ingredients

8-ounce packet of cream cheese, softened

1½ cups cauliflower rice

½ teaspoon Worcestershire sauce

1 tablespoon onion powder

1 teaspoon garlic

1 teaspoon ginger

4 ounces grated pepperjack cheese

¼ cup grated Parmesan cheese

Salt and pepper to taste

¼ cup everything bagel seasoning

Savory Mini Meat Pies

ingredients

For the crust: (if you'd rather, you can substitute premade pie crust)

3 cups flour

1 teaspoon salt

1¼ cups shortening

1 egg

5 tablespoons water

1 tablespoon vinegar

For the filling:

2 tablespoons unsalted butter

½ cup diced leeks or onion

2 cloves garlic, minced

1½ pound ground beef

⅔ cup red wine
or ¾ cup tomato sauce

½ cup riced carrots

¼ cup riced broccoli

½ cup minced celery

1 teaspoon pepper

½ teaspoon salt

1 teaspoon curry powder

½ teaspoon chili powder

1 tablespoon dried oregano

1 tablespoon basic

2 teaspoons dried rosemary

2 eggs

⅔ cup Parmesan cheese

directions: crust

1. In a large bowl, add all the ingredients for the pie crust.
2. Blend using a pastry cutter or your hands until a soft dough forms.
3. Lightly flour a work surface and roll out the dough to about ¼-inch thickness.
4. Using a 3-inch round cutter, cut out dough circles for your pies.
5. Place on a parchment-lined baking sheet and set aside.

directions: filling

1. Melt butter in a large skillet over medium heat.
2. Add the leeks or onion with minced garlic and sauté for 3 to 4 minutes.
3. Add the ground beef and cook until no longer pink.
4. Drain fat if necessary.
5. Add wine and simmer for 2 to 3 minutes.
6. Reduce heat to low and add the spices, carrot, broccoli, and celery. Simmer for 15 minutes.
7. Remove from heat and add the Parmesan cheese and one egg. Mix well then set aside.

assembling

8. In a small bowl, beat the second egg with one tablespoon of water for the egg wash. Set aside.
9. Fill half of each prepared dough circle with the meat mixture, leaving a clean edge of dough on the outside. Lightly moisten one edge of the dough with water and fold over, pressing the edges to seal.
10. Deep fry in 375°F oil for 2 to 3 minutes.
11. Drain on a paper towel and serve hot.

IDEA: *Makes a Great Main Dish too!* Use a 4- to 6-inch round cutter for larger pies. Add an egg wash to the tops, then bake at 425°F for 25 to 30 minutes. Use a biscuit cutter to make smaller circles. Fill as directed, then deep fry at 375°F for 4 to 6 minutes, flipping over after 2 to 3 minutes per side.

Bacon Spinach Pesto Roll-Ups

directions

1. In a large bowl, combine the **spinach purée** and pesto.

2. Roll out the pizza crust into a large rectangle.

3. Spread the pesto–spinach blend on top of the crust.

4. Sprinkle with red pepper, bacon, and mozzarella cheese.

5. Starting from the widest side, roll the dough up into a large log and wrap it in plastic wrap.

6. Refrigerate for 30 minutes or until firm.

7. Preheat oven to 400°F.

8. Line a large baking sheet with parchment paper.

9. Remove the refrigerated roll, remove plastic wrap and place roll on a clean work surface.

10. Starting at one end, slice into 1- to 2-inch thick slices.

11. Place each slice flat (pinwheel side up) on the prepared baking sheet.

12. Sprinkle the top of each piece with shredded cheese.

13. Bake for 15 to 20 minutes or until lightly browned.

Tip: Try a different twist! Use a homemade **Kale & Pea Pesto** from page 58 is place of the jar of pesto.

ingredients

One 6.25 ounce jar of pesto

½ cup **spinach purée**

1 premade refrigerated pizza crust

½ teaspoon crushed red pepper

1 cup crumbled bacon pieces

1 cup shredded mozzarella cheese

½ cup shredded Gruyere or other Swiss cheese

Battered Spicy Cauliflower Bites

ingredients: dipping sauce

¾ cup rice vinegar

½ cup sugar

1½ teaspoons red chili pepper flakes

1½ teaspoons salt

1½ large garlic clove, minced

ingredients: batter

½ cup cornstarch

½ cup flour

½ teaspoon baking powder

⅓ cup toasted sesame seeds (may substitute sunflower kernels or poppy seeds)

⅓ cup unsweetened coconut flakes

½ cup cold water

½ cup vodka

1 head cauliflower, cut into 1-inch florets

sesame oil for frying

directions

1. Cut cauliflower into 1-inch florets. Set aside.

2. To make the sauce: Combine all of the sauce ingredients in a small saucepan. Cook on medium heat, stirring with a wooden spoon until the sugar dissolves. Increase the heat to medium-high and let boil for 5 to 10 minutes or so, until the mixture becomes syrupy. Remove from heat and let cool. The sauce should continue to thicken as it cools.

3. Heat oil to 350°F in a large wok, pan, or deep fryer.

4. While the sauce is heating, combine the dry batter ingredients in a large bowl and whisk. Mix in the water and vodka to make a thin batter.

5. Drop cauliflower florets into the batter, a few pieces at a time. Flip to coat completely. Using tongs, remove the cauliflower one floret at a time from the batter and shake to remove excess batter.

6. Place the florets in the hot oil until the pan or fryer is full but not overcrowded.

7. Cook for about 3 minutes until the coated florets are crisp and golden brown.

8. Remove and drain off the oil on a paper towel. Continue until all the pieces are cooked.

9. Drizzle with dipping sauce and serve.

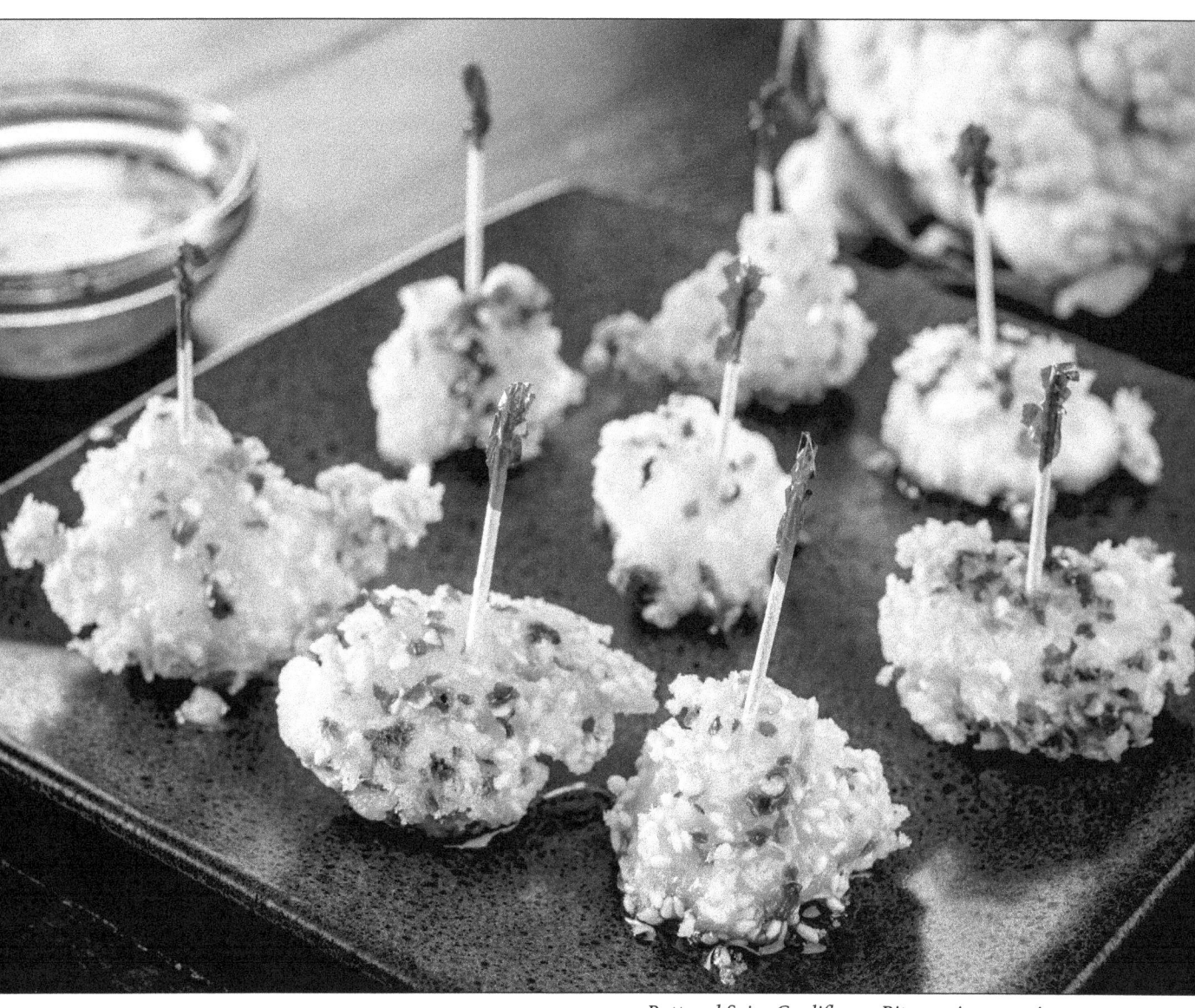

Battered Spicy Cauliflower Bites; recipe opposite page

© Scott Erb & Donna Dufault – www.erbphoto.com

Veggie Poppers

ingredients

½ cup raspberry vinaigrette dressing

¼ cup mayonnaise

1 cup riced cauliflower

1 cup riced broccoli

1 cup riced carrot

1 cup plain, dry bread crumbs

½ cup grated Parmesan cheese

directions

1. Preheat oven to 425° F. Line a baking sheet with parchment paper.

2. In a large bowl, whisk vinaigrette dressing and mayonnaise until smooth.

3. Add the riced cauliflower, broccoli, and carrots, bread crumbs, and grated Parmesan cheese, mixing until just blended.

4. Roll the mix into balls and place on the baking sheet.

5. Bake for 25-30 minutes or until the poppers are crisp on the outside.

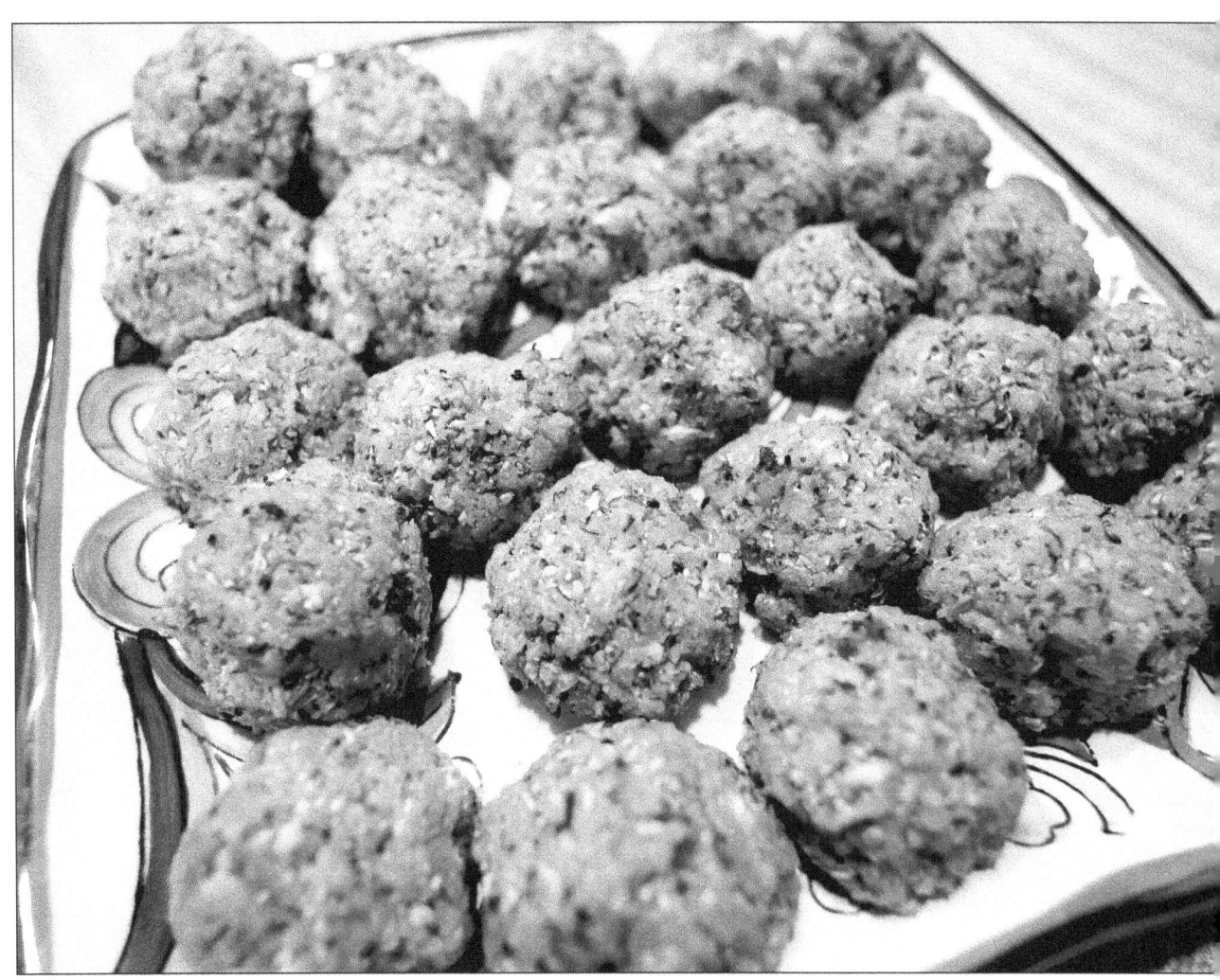

Veggie Crust Mini Pizza

directions

1. Turn on the broiler.

2. Split the spinach buns and lay them out, cut side up, on the baking sheet.

3. Toast the buns in the broiler for 2 to 3 minutes until lightly browned. Remove and set aside.

4. Preheat oven to 350°F.

5. Cook the ground beef for about 10 minutes in a large skillet over medium heat, until browned and crumbly.

6. Drain any excess grease and return to heat.

7. Add leeks or onions, carrots, and **bell peppers.** Cook for about 5 minutes until the vegetables are softened.

8. Add the Italian seasoning, garlic powder, onion powder, crushed red pepper flakes, and paprika, blending well.

9. Add pizza sauce and Parmesan cheese and bring to a boil.

10. Reduce heat and simmer for 10 to 15 minutes, stirring often.

11. Remove from heat.

12. Spoon the beef mixture over the prepared buns.

13. Top each bun with about ¼ cup of the shredded mozzarella cheese.

14. Bake for about 10 minutes, until the cheese is bubbly and lightly browned.

ingredients

8 spinach hamburger buns, split (see recipe on p. 80)

1 lb of ground beef

⅓ cup minced leeks or onion

¼ cup riced carrots

¼ cup **minced red bell pepper**

2¼ teaspoons Italian seasoning

1 teaspoon garlic powder

¼ teaspoon onion powder

⅛ teaspoon crushed red pepper flakes

1 teaspoon paprika

One 15-ounce can of pizza sauce

⅓ cup grated Parmesan cheese

2 cups shredded mozzarella cheese

Tangy Meatballs

ingredients: sauce

½ cup barbeque sauce

1 cup ketchup

2 tablespoons white or apple cider vinegar

1 teaspoon chili powder

1 teaspoon yellow mustard

¼ cup brown sugar

ingredients: meatballs

1 lb ground beef

1 large egg, beaten

¼ cup breadcrumbs

¼ cup finely diced onion

½ cup riced carrot

½ cup riced broccoli

2 teaspoons minced garlic

¾ teaspoon salt

¼ teaspoon ground black pepper

directions

1. Preheat the oven to 400°F.

2. Line a baking sheet with foil and spray with non-stick cooking spray.

3. In a medium-sized bowl, blend all the sauce ingredients with a spoon. Set aside.

4. In a large bowl, add all the ingredients for the meatballs. Mix well using a spoon or with your hands.

5. Form 1-inch balls from the meat mixture. Place on the prepared baking sheet. Spoon a small amount of sauce over each meatball to cover completely. Reserve any remaining sauce for serving.

6. Bake for 18 to 20 minutes.

IDEA: *Makes a Great Main Dish too!* Shape the mix into 1½- to 2-inch-sized meatballs. When cooked, serve with sauce over rice or mashed potatoes. Busy day? Make ahead and cook in the crockpot on low with the entire quantity of sauce.

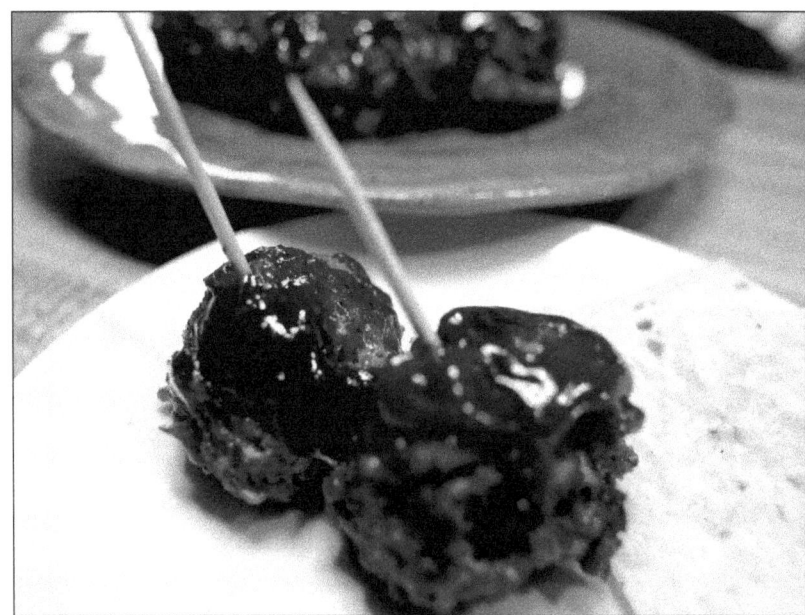

Potato Broccoli Soup

directions

1. Cook the bacon in a large soup pot over medium heat until crisp and browned. Remove and drain on a clean paper towel.

2. Add butter and diced leeks or onion to the pot. Cook for about 3 minutes until translucent.

3. Add diced potatoes, broccoli, chicken broth, milk, heavy cream, chili powder, salt, and pepper. Stir well.

4. Bring to a boil.

5. Lower heat to simmer and cook for about 15 minutes or until the potatoes are tender.

6. Keep the pot on the stovetop, but remove from direct heat.

7. Using a potato masher, carefully crush potato chunks until the soup reaches the desired consistency. Stir with a wire whisk to blend.

8. Return to heat and simmer for 10 minutes.

9. When serving, top with sour cream, bacon, cheddar cheese, and chives.

ingredients

3 strips bacon

2 tablespoons butter

2 cups diced leeks or onion

4 large gold potatoes, peeled and diced

½ cup minced broccoli

2 cups chicken broth

1 cup milk

½ cup heavy cream

½ tablespoon chili powder

1 teaspoon salt

1 teaspoon pepper

Optional toppings to serve:
   sour cream
   crumbled bacon
   cheddar cheese
   chives

Easy Vegetable Soup

ingredients

4–6 cups water

3 tablespoons vegetable bouillon powder

2 15.5 ounce cans diced tomatoes

2 cups diced leeks or onion

2/3 cup diced celery

1½ cups diced carrots

2 15.5 ounce cans pinto beans

½ cup diced broccoli

2/3 cup **shredded zucchini**
   (or 1 small zucchini, sliced thin)

2 cups diced red pepper

½ cup riced Brussels sprouts

Salt to taste

Pepper to taste

1 teaspoon chili powder

2 teaspoons garlic powder

1 teaspoon cilantro

1 tablespoon parsley

1 bay leaf

directions

1. Add all the ingredients to a large stockpot.

2. Bring to a boil.

3. Reduce heat and simmer for 2 to 3 hours.

IDEA: *Make it Meaty!* Add 1 lb of cooked ground beef, Italian sausage, sliced smoked sausage, or chicken.

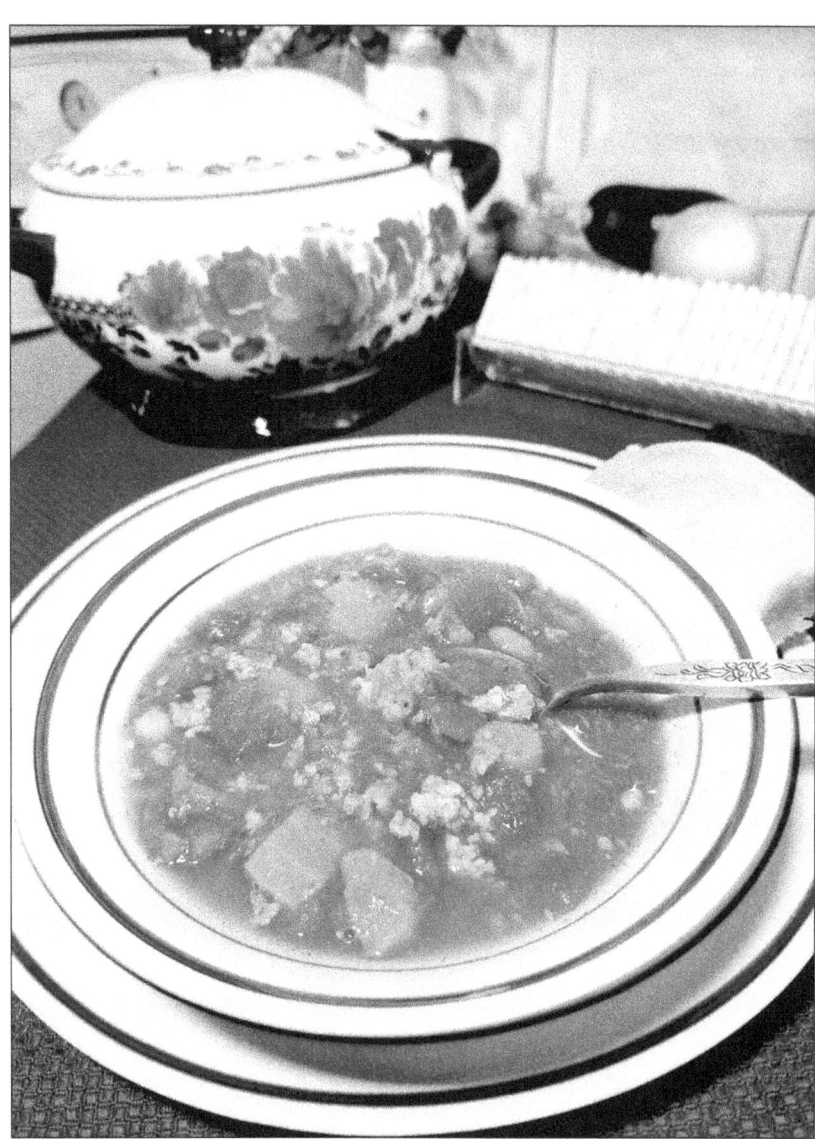

Slow Cooker Tortellini Kale Soup

directions

1. Brown sausage in a large frying pan or saucepan. Drain any fat.

2. Add garlic and leeks or onion and cook for 4 to 6 minutes, or until soft.

3. In a crockpot or slow cooker, combine the **tomatoes**, chicken broth, water, red wine, **puréed kale,** and dried tortellini.

4. Add the sausage, garlic, and leeks or onions.

5. Cook on low for 4 hours.

ingredients

1 lb of ground hot Italian sausage

2 garlic cloves, diced

2 cups diced leeks or onions

One 28-ounce can of crushed or **diced tomatoes**

4 cups chicken broth

1 cup water

½ cup dry red wine

½ cup **puréed kale**

One 12-ounce package of dried three-cheese tortellini

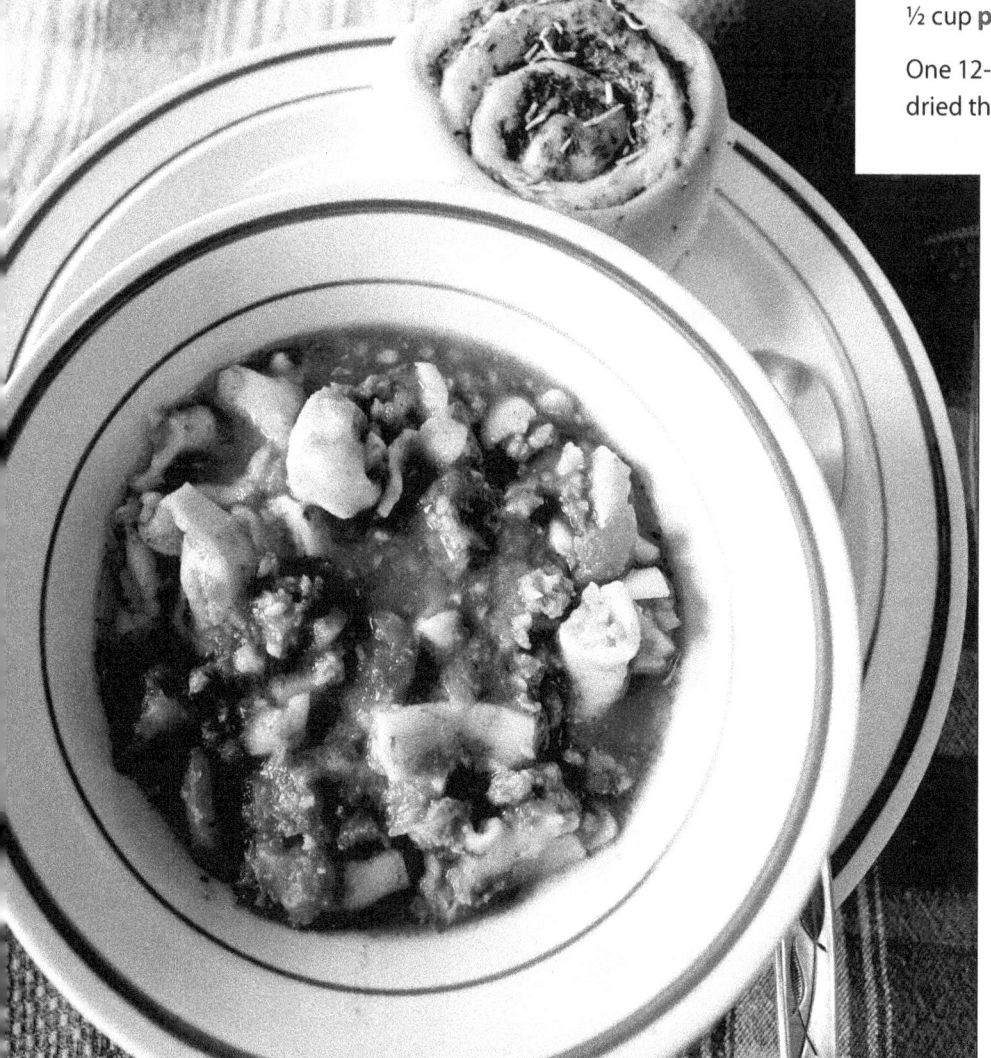

Appetizers, Soups & Snacks

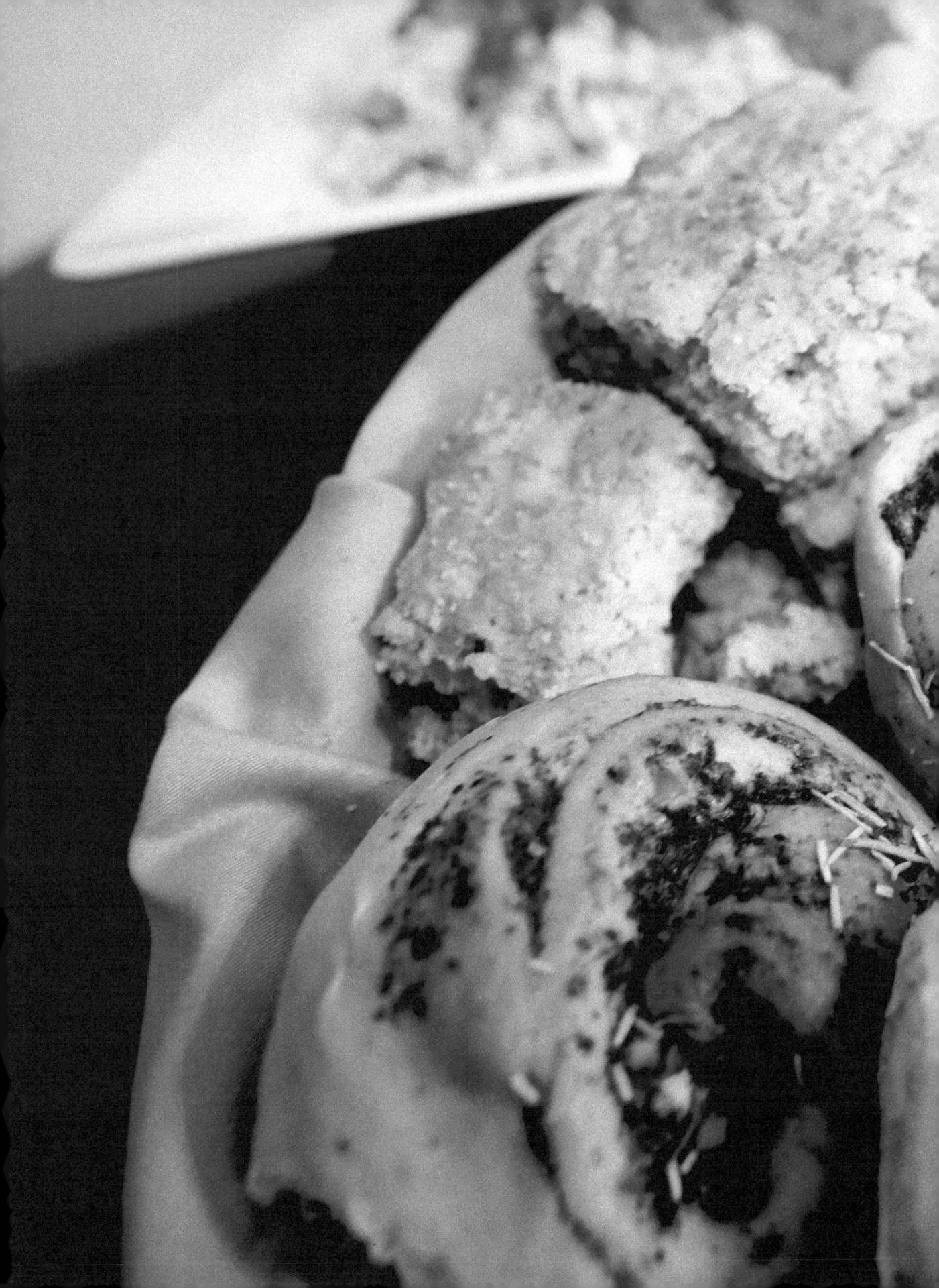

Breads

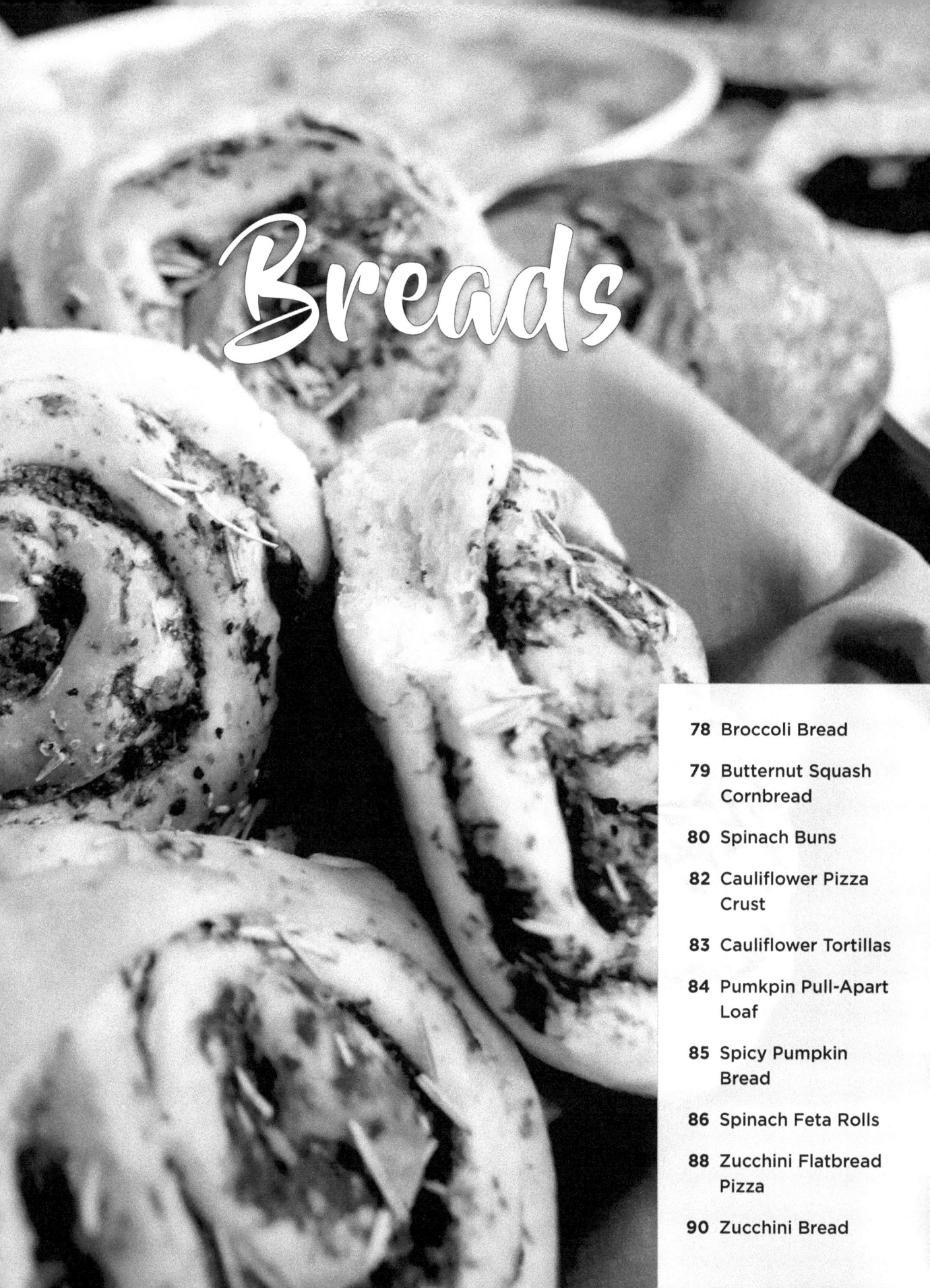

- 78 Broccoli Bread
- 79 Butternut Squash Cornbread
- 80 Spinach Buns
- 82 Cauliflower Pizza Crust
- 83 Cauliflower Tortillas
- 84 Pumkpin Pull-Apart Loaf
- 85 Spicy Pumpkin Bread
- 86 Spinach Feta Rolls
- 88 Zucchini Flatbread Pizza
- 90 Zucchini Bread

Broccoli Bread

ingredients

2 cups riced broccoli

8 eggs

1 cup breadcrumbs

½ teaspoon salt

directions

1. Preheat oven to 400°F.
2. Line a 9x13 baking sheet with parchment paper.
3. In a medium bowl, mix riced broccoli, eggs, breadcrumbs, and salt until well blended.
4. Spoon the batter onto the tray and press firmly to spread evenly until approximately ⅓-inch thick.
5. Bake for 20 to 25 minutes or until the bread is slightly browned and firm to the touch.
6. Cool the tray on a wire rack.
7. Cut the bread into equal pieces.

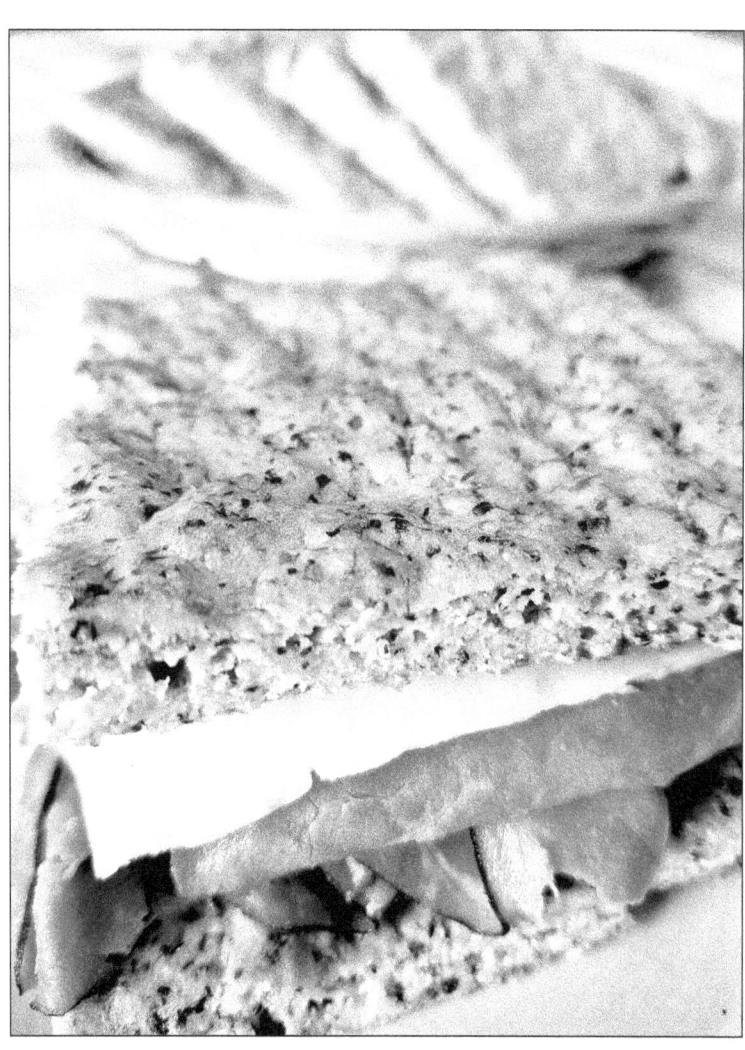

Butternut Squash Cornbread

directions

1. Preheat oven to 350°F.
2. Spray an 8x8 pan with non-stick cooking spray.
3. In a medium bowl, whisk together the flour, cornmeal, baking powder, baking soda, and salt.
4. In a large bowl, mix the melted butter with brown sugar. Add egg, butternut squash purée, and buttermilk. Mix until just blended.
5. Slowly add the flour mixture to the squash purée mix and stir with a wooden spoon until just combined.
6. Pour the batter into the prepared pan.
7. Bake for between 45 minutes to an hour.
8. Cool on a wire rack.

ingredients

1 cup of all-purpose flour

1 cup cornmeal

2 teaspoons baking powder

½ teaspoon baking soda

⅛ teaspoon salt

⅓ cup unsalted butter, melted

¼ cup brown sugar

1 egg

⅓ cup puréed butternut squash

¾ cup buttermilk (or whole milk)

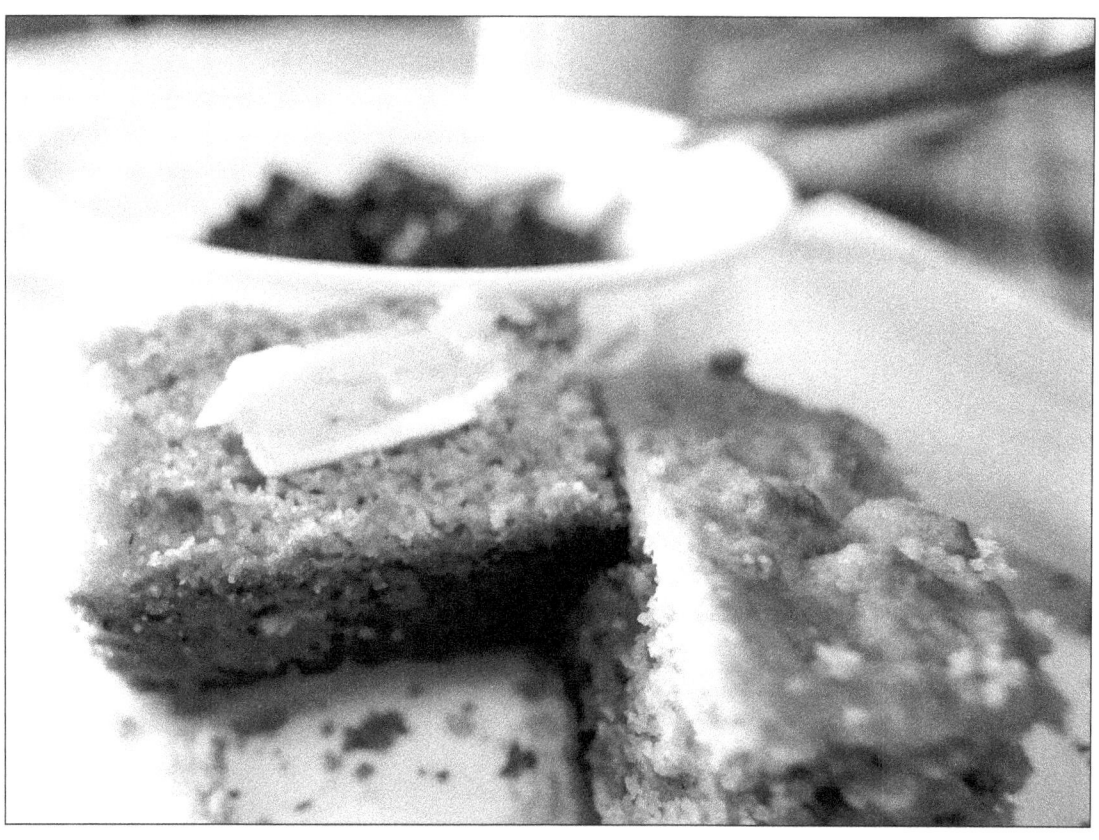

Spinach Buns

ingredients

3–3¼ cups all-purpose flour

2 teaspoons instant yeast

½ cup milk at room temperature

1 egg

1 teaspoon salt

1 cup **spinach purée**

2 tablespoons vegetable oil

Sesame seeds (optional)

directions

1. In a large bowl, whisk the flour, yeast, and salt.

2. Add milk, egg, **spinach purée,** and vegetable oil. Use a wooden spoon or your hands to mix well.

3. On a clean, lightly floured surface, knead 8 to 10 times only to blend.

4. Lightly grease a large glass or ceramic bowl (yeast will not rise as well in plastic). Place the dough in the bowl and cover with a clean towel. Set in a warm, draft-free location for 45 to 60 minutes, or until the dough has doubled in volume.

5. Line a baking sheet with parchment paper and lightly spray with cooking oil.

6. Punch the dough gently to deflate, then turn it out on a clean, lightly floured surface.

7. Cut the dough into eight equal pieces.

8. Roll each piece into a ball, then pat to slightly flatten the top, forming the bun shape.

9. Place on the baking sheet, with at least a 2-inch gap between the buns.

10. Cover and allow to set in a warm, draft-free location for 30 minutes, or until the buns have almost doubled in size. The buns may nearly touch now but should not be connected.

11. Brush the rolls with butter and sprinkle with sesame seeds.

12. Preheat the oven to 375°F.

13. Bake for 18 to 20 minutes. The seeds should be lightly browned and the texture of each roll firm.

14. Remove the buns from the oven and cool on a wire rack for 5 minutes before cutting and serving.

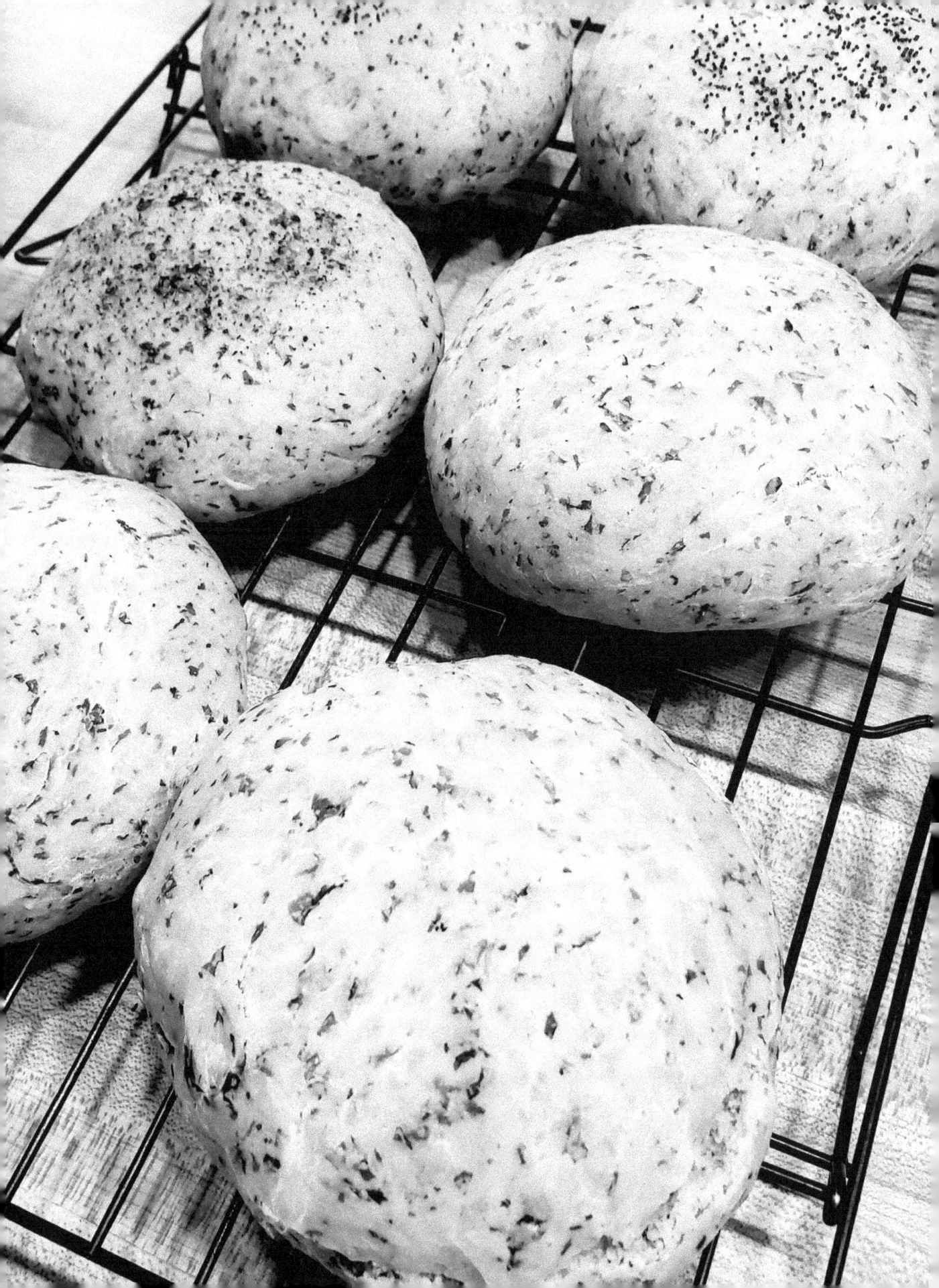

Cauliflower Pizza Crust

ingredients

2 cups riced cauliflower

¼ teaspoon onion powder

¼ teaspoon garlic powder

1 egg (if small, add enough water to equal ¼ cup liquid)

1 cup grated Parmesan cheese

Pizza sauce

Shredded mozzarella cheese

Your favorite pizza toppings like pepperoni or sausage

Photo opposite page

directions

1. Preheat oven to 400°F.

2. Line a baking sheet with parchment paper and lightly spray with cooking oil.

3. In a dry skillet over medium heat, spread the riced cauliflower, onion powder, and garlic powder.

4. Using a spatula to turn occasionally, heat for about 10 minutes until the mixture looks dry, but not toasted or burned.

5. Add grated Parmesan cheese and continue to cook on medium heat until the cheese is melted.

6. Remove from the heat and stir in the egg.

7. Divide the dough in half.

8. Place the first section of dough on the parchment paper. Form into a 12-inch round crust, building it up slightly on the edges for a crust, but keeping the center thickness uniform and level (Do not allow the center to become too thin or your crust won't hold the toppings).

9. Repeat with the remaining dough.

10. Bake for 20 minutes, then remove from oven, but maintain oven temperature.

11. Top each pizza with sauce, mozzarella cheese, and your favorite toppings.

12. Return to the oven and bake for another 10 minutes.

13. Cool for 5 minutes before cutting.

14. Serve warm.

Cauliflower Tortillas

directions

1. Preheat oven to 375°F.

2. Line a baking sheet with parchment paper and lightly spray with cooking oil.

3. In a large bowl, combine the riced cauliflower, eggs, oregano, paprika, salt, and pepper until blended.

4. Form the dough into 6 equal balls.

5. Place the balls on the parchment paper and press to flatten each one into a circle.

6. Bake for 8 to 10 minutes.

7. Remove from oven, turn each tortilla over, then return to the oven and bake for an additional 5 minutes.

8. Serve warm. Makes great quesadillas!

9. Store leftovers in the refrigerator. Reheat in a skillet over medium heat for 1 to 2 minutes.

ingredients

4 cups riced cauliflower

2 large eggs

½ teaspoon dried oregano

½ teaspoon paprika

½ teaspoon salt

½ teaspoon freshly ground black pepper

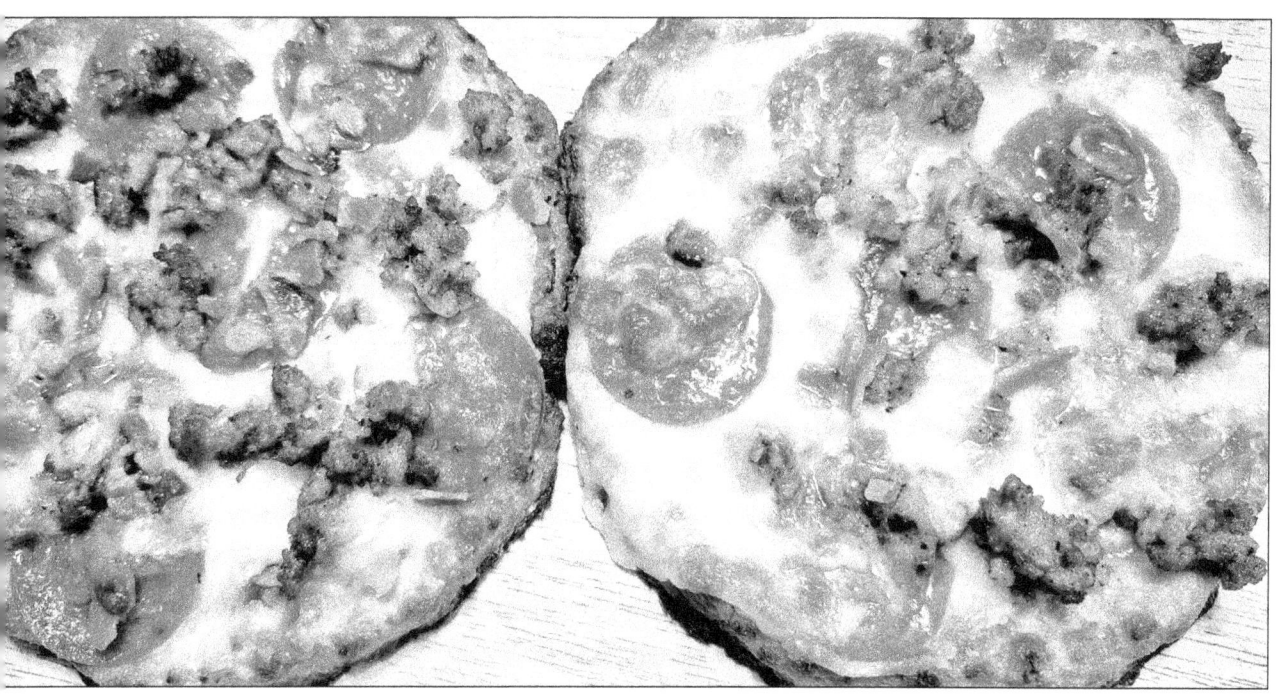

Cauliflower Crust Pizza recipe opposite page.

Pumpkin Pull-Apart Loaf

ingredients

- ¾ cup pumpkin purée
- 1 egg
- 1 teaspoon vanilla extract
- 1 teaspoon pumpkin pie spice
- ½ cup granulated sugar, divided
- One 8-count packet of ready-to-bake biscuits
- 1 cup ground walnuts
- 2 teaspoons cinnamon, divided
- ½ cup powdered sugar
- 3 tablespoons heavy whipping cream or milk

directions

1. Preheat oven to 350°F. Spray a 9x5 loaf pan with nonstick cooking spray.
2. In a medium bowl, combine pumpkin purée, egg, vanilla extract, cinnamon, pumpkin pie spice, and ¼ cup granulated sugar.
3. In a small bowl, whisk the remaining ¼ cup of granulated sugar with 1 teaspoon of cinnamon.
4. Remove the biscuit dough from the container and place on a clean cutting board. Cut each biscuit into four equal pieces.
5. Toss the wedges of biscuit dough with the cinnamon–sugar mixture to coat completely.
6. Lay enough pieces of dough to cover the bottom of the loaf pan.
7. Spread ⅓ of the pumpkin mixture, then sprinkle ⅓ of the ground walnuts on top.
8. Add two more layers of dough, pumpkin, and walnuts.
9. Bake for 20 to 25 minutes, or until the top is golden and the center is cooked through.
10. Cool on a wire rack for 10 minutes.
11. Remove the loaf from the pan by covering the pan with a plate and flipping. Turn over on the plate to glaze.
12. *To make the glaze:* Whisk the powdered sugar, remaining 1 teaspoon of cinnamon, and heavy whipping cream until smooth. Drizzle over pumpkin loaf before serving.

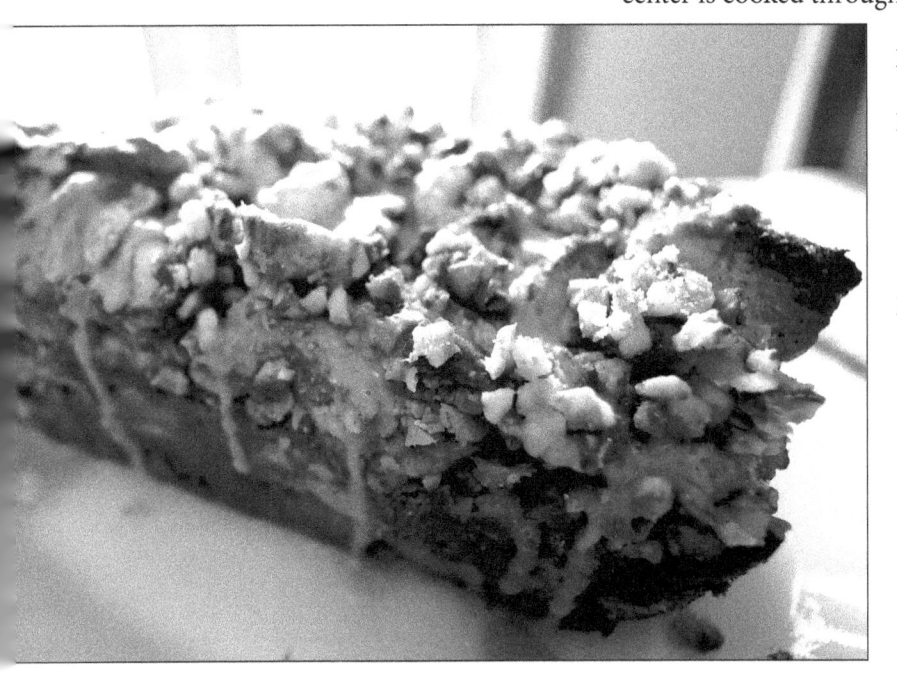

Spicy Pumpkin Bread

directions

1. Preheat oven to 350°F.
2. Spray two 9x5 bread loaf pans with non-stick cooking spray.
3. In a large bowl, combine flour, allspice, cinnamon, nutmeg, cloves, salt, and baking soda.
4. In a medium bowl, combine brown sugar, milk, eggs, **beet purée,** pumpkin purée, and vanilla extract. Stir to combine.
5. Add the pumpkin mixture to the flour mixture, stirring until just moist.
6. Fold in walnuts.
7. Pour the batter into prepared pans.
8. Bake at 350°F for 1 hour or until a wooden pick inserted in the loaf's center comes out clean.
9. Cool in the pans for 10 minutes on a wire rack, then remove from the pans.
10. Cool completely.

ingredients

3½ cups all-purpose flour

2 teaspoons baking powder

1 teaspoon ground allspice

1 teaspoon ground cinnamon

1 teaspoon ground nutmeg

½ teaspoon ground cloves

¾ teaspoon salt

½ teaspoon baking soda

1⅓ cups packed brown sugar

¾ cup milk

2 large eggs

⅓ cup **beet purée**

2 cups pumpkin purée

2 teaspoons vanilla extract

⅓ cup chopped walnuts

Spinach Feta Rolls

ingredients: dough

1 cup milk

2¼ teaspoons active dry yeast

2 tablespoons sugar

4 tablespoons unsalted butter, melted

1 egg yolk

2¾ cups all-purpose flour

1 teaspoon salt

ingredients: filling

4 tablespoons unsalted butter, plus 2 tablespoons at room temperature for the pan

2 tablespoons minced leeks or onion

1½ cup **spinach purée**

½ cup crumbled feta

¼ cup grated Parmesan

¼ teaspoon nutmeg

½ teaspoon lemon pepper

ingredients: topping

4 tablespoons unsalted butter

1 tablespoon dried rosemary

1 teaspoon lemon pepper

directions

1. Heat milk for 30 to 45 seconds in a small microwave-safe bowl. The liquid should be warm, not hot.

2. Add yeast and 1 teaspoon sugar. Whisk lightly to blend and allow to sit for about 5 minutes until foamy.

3. Add the 4 tablespoons of melted and cooled butter and the egg yolk, whisking to combine.

4. Add flour, salt, and remaining sugar.

5. Mix well by hand until the dough comes together.

6. Turn onto a floured surface and knead until soft and elastic.

7. Lightly coat the inside of a large glass or ceramic bowl with olive oil. Place the dough in the bowl, turning once to coat the dough with oil.

8. Cover the bowl with plastic wrap and place in a warm, draft-free location. Allow the dough to rise for 60 to 90 minutes or until it doubles in volume.

9. To prepare the filling, melt the butter in a skillet over medium heat.

10. Add the chopped leeks or onion and cook until soft and translucent. Remove from heat and allow to cool.

11. In a medium bowl, combine the **spinach purée,** feta, Parmesan, nutmeg, and lemon pepper. Add the cooled leeks. Mix well.

12. Refrigerate the filling mixture, if necessary, until the dough has risen sufficiently.

13. When the dough has doubled, punch down lightly and let it rest for 1 to 2 minutes.

14. Line a baking pan at least 2-inches deep with parchment paper and lightly spray with cooking oil.

15. Lightly flour a clean, flat surface like a kitchen counter or table. Roll out the dough to approximately 18x24.

16. Spread the filling evenly over the dough, leaving a 1-inch strip of dough untouched.

17. Roll the dough into a tight log, finishing with the plain dough at the bottom to seal the edges together.

Spinach Feta Rolls (continued)

18. Slice the log into about 12 equal-inch rolls and place in the prepared pan so that the pinwheel design is facing up.

19. Cover the pan with plastic wrap and allow rolls to rise for about 60 minutes or until they double in volume.

20. Preheat to 350°F.

21. Bake the rolls for 25 to 30 minutes or until lightly browned.

22. Remove and set them on racks to cool.

23. Melt the 4 tablespoons of butter in a small microwave-safe bowl. Add rosemary and lemon pepper and whisk lightly to blend. Brush the mixture over the rolls.

24. Serve warm.

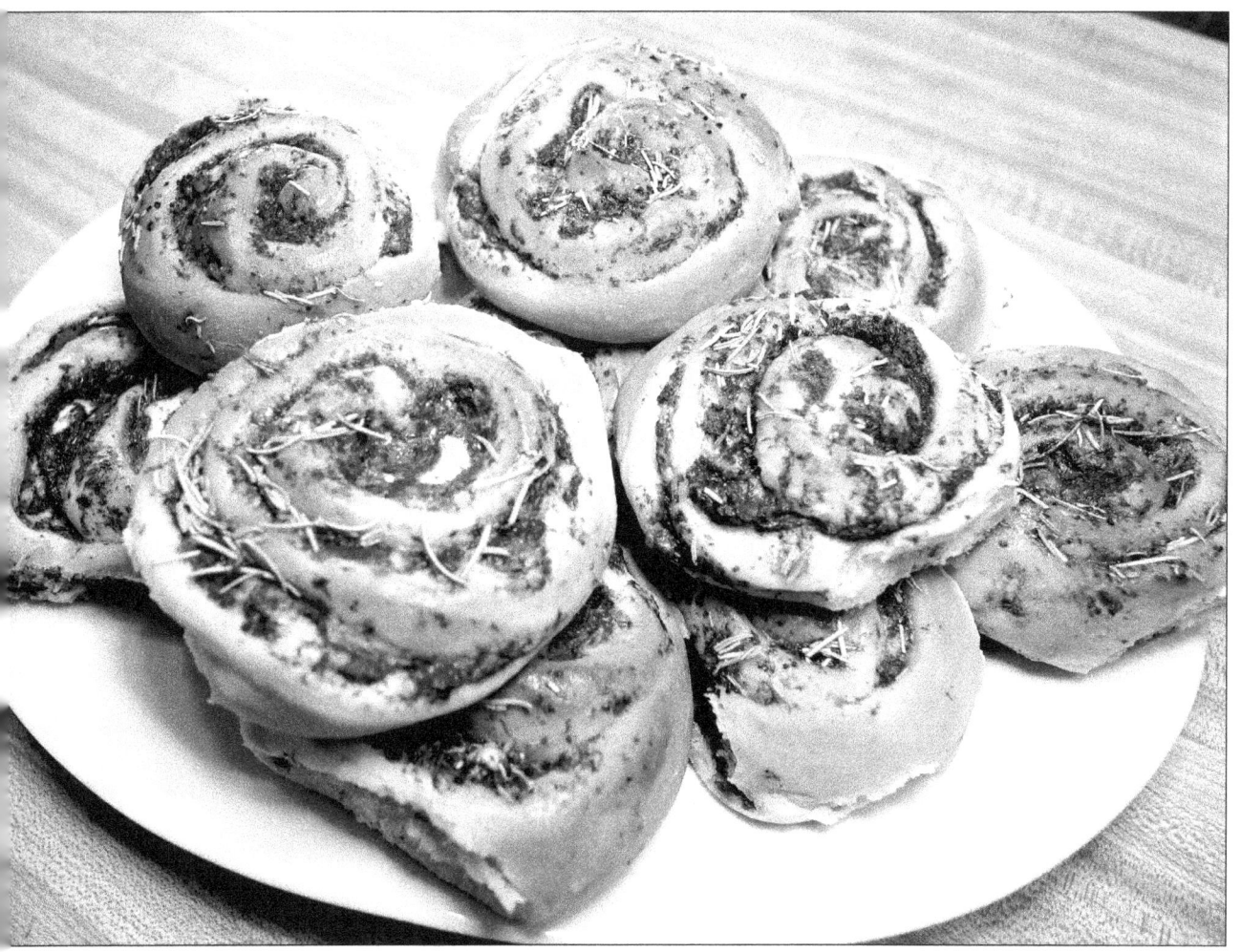

Zucchini Flatbread Pizza

ingredients: dough

1½ teaspoons active dry yeast

1 teaspoon granulated sugar

¾ cup warm water (about 100°F)

2 cups all-purpose flour

1 tablespoon olive oil

1 teaspoon salt

ingredients: topping

2 cups **roasted cherry tomatoes**

2 cups shredded zucchini

½ cup Ricotta cheese

½ teaspoon rosemary

½ teaspoon granulated garlic

1 teaspoon olive oil

4 ounces pepperjack cheese

4 ounces of crumbled feta or blue cheese

Pepperoni, Italian sausage, ham, bacon, or other pizza toppings

directions

1. In a small bowl, whisk yeast and sugar with warm water. The liquid should be warm, but not hot. Whisk 2 to 3 circles to blend. Allow to sit for about 5 minutes until foamy.

2. Add flour, olive oil, and salt. Beat by hand or on low speed with a mixer until the ingredients are mixed well. The dough should be thick and shaggy.

3. Transfer it to a lightly floured work surface. Knead for 3 to 4 minutes until it becomes soft and elastic. The dough should be soft and pliable; work in small amounts of flour as needed to reduce stickiness.

4. Lightly grease a large glass or ceramic bowl (yeast will not rise as well in plastic). Place the dough in the bowl and cover with a clean towel. Set in a warm, draft-free location for 45 to 60 minutes or until the dough has doubled in volume.

5. Mix the Ricotta, rosemary, and garlic in a medium bowl until smooth. Cover and refrigerate.

6. When the dough has risen, preheat the oven to 475°F.

7. Place shredded zucchini in a colander in the sink to allow any excess moisture to drain.

8. Prepare two sheets of parchment paper, roughly half the size of your baking sheet. The flatbreads will get cooked side by side. You can use two small baking sheets as well.

9. Separate the dough into two equal parts.

10. Place the first piece of parchment paper on a countertop or table. Transfer one portion of the dough onto it and roll it into a rectangle about ¼-inch thick. Transfer the parchment onto the baking sheet. Repeat with the second portion of dough.

11. Using a fork, prick a few holes into the surface of the dough and drizzle with a ½ teaspoon of olive oil for each portion of dough.

12. Spread half of the Ricotta mixture on each dough portion. Add a uniform layer of shredded zucchini and **tomatoes**.

13. Sprinkle with feta and top with mozzarella. Add your favorite pizza toppings.

14. Bake for 15 to 20 minutes or until the crust and toppings are browned. Remove from the oven.

15. Allow the pizza to sit for 1 to 2 minutes before cutting. Serve warm.

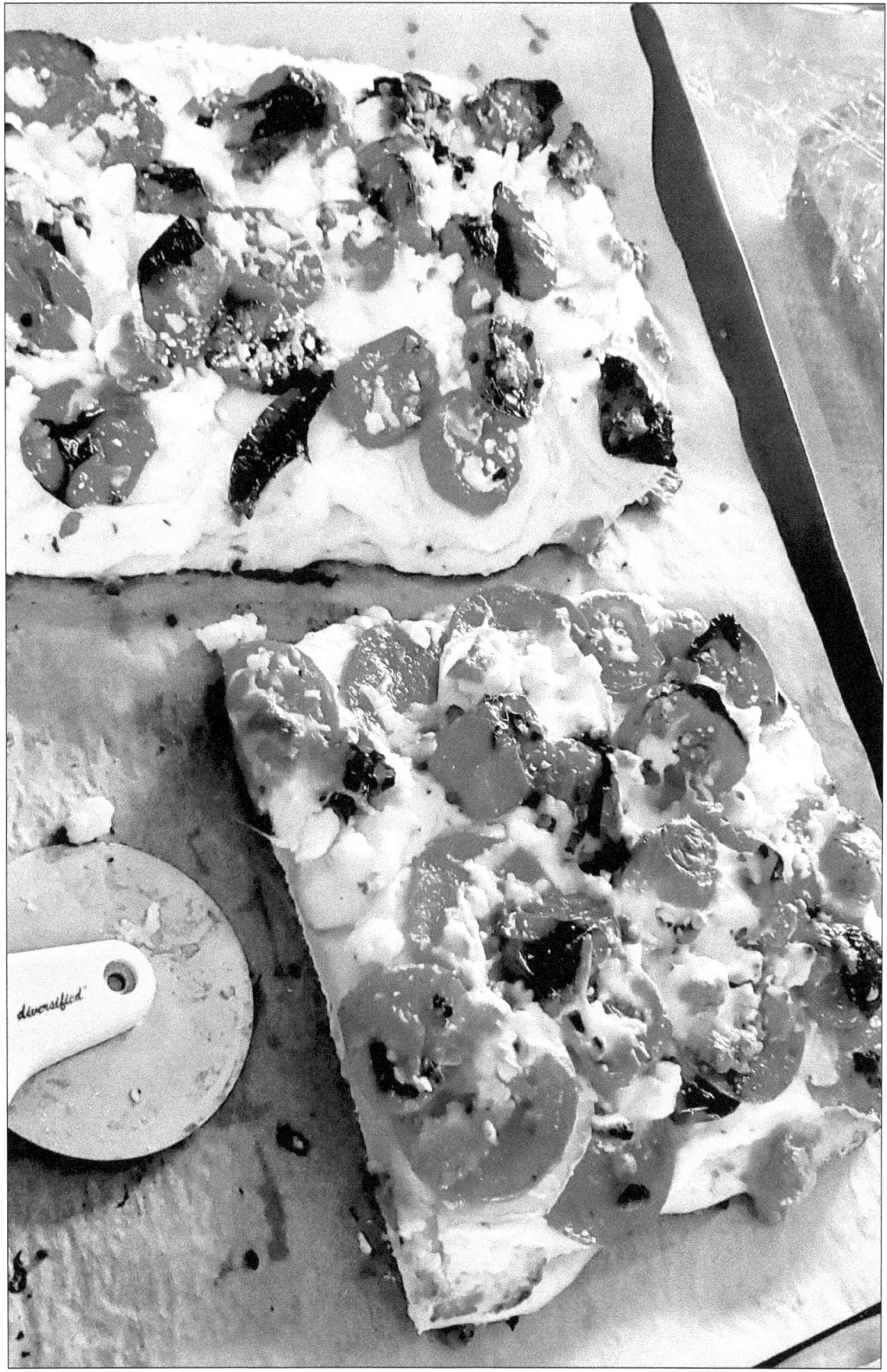

Zucchini Bread

ingredients

3 cups all-purpose flour

1 teaspoon salt

1 teaspoon baking soda

1 teaspoon baking powder

1 tablespoon ground cinnamon

3 eggs

1 cup plain or vanilla-flavored yogurt

2¼ cups sugar

3 teaspoons vanilla extract

2 cups **shredded zucchini**

1 cup chopped walnuts

directions

1. Preheat oven to 325°F.
2. Spray two 9x5 loaf pans with nonstick cooking spray.
3. In a large bowl, blend the eggs, yogurt, sugar, and vanilla.
4. In a medium bowl, whisk flour, salt, baking powder, baking soda, and cinnamon until blended.
5. Gradually add the flour mixture to the large bowl, blending until fully incorporated.
6. Fold in **zucchini** and nuts until fully mixed.
7. Divide the batter equally between the prepared pans.
8. Bake for 50 to 60 minutes or until the tester inserted into the dough's center comes out clean.
9. Remove from the oven and cool on a wire rack for 15 minutes before removing the bread from the pans.

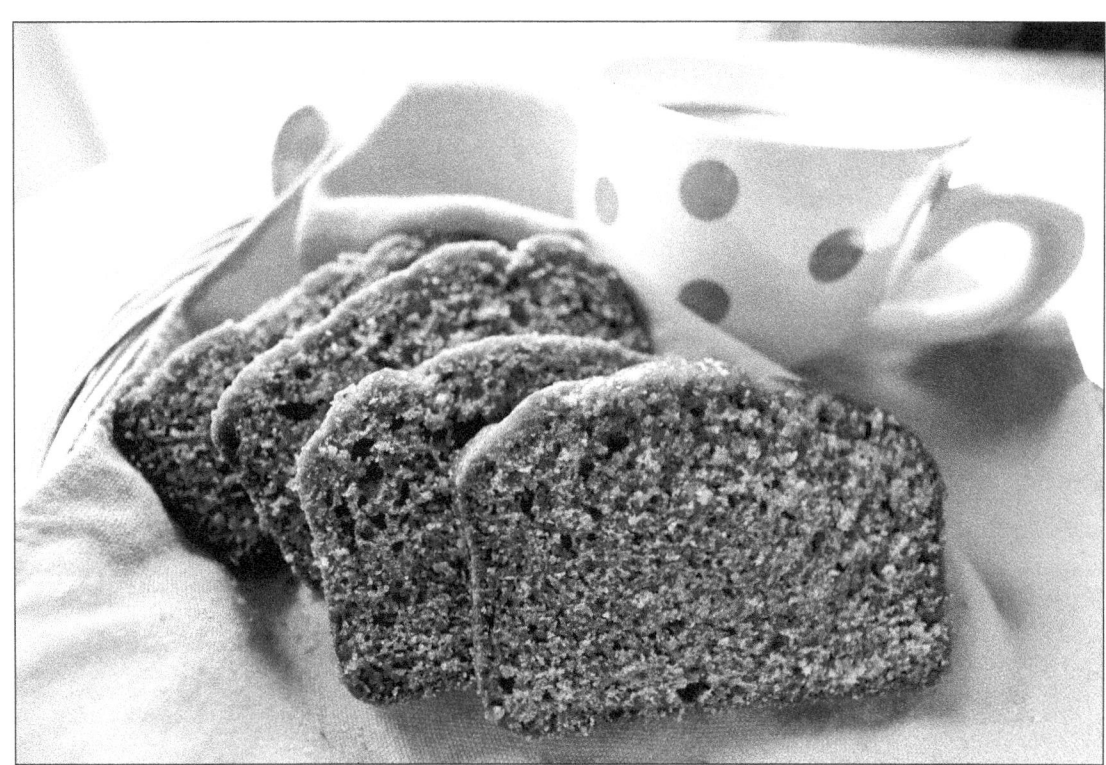

Breakfast

- 92 Carrot Coffeecake Muffins
- 94 Asparagus Frittata
- 95 Sausage and Chard Frittata
- 96 Breakfast Turnovers
- 97 Nutty Egg Waffles
- 98 Morning Potato Nachos
- 100 Bacon and Cheese Quiche
- 101 Crockpot Breakfast Casserole
- 102 Glazed Beet Donuts
- 104 Banana Cauliflower Muffins
- 105 Pumpkin-Cranberry Muffins
- 106 Omelet Muffins

Carrot Coffeecake Muffins

ingredients: cake

2 cups flour

2½ teaspoons baking powder

1 teaspoon salt

1½ teaspoons cinnamon

½ teaspoon pumpkin pie spice

½ cup butter (room temperature)

1 cup brown sugar

1 cup granulated sugar

2 eggs

1 tablespoon vanilla

1 cup buttermilk

2½ cups riced carrots

1 cup sweetened shredded coconut

ingredients: cream cheese filling

8 ounces cream cheese (room temperature)

¼ cup granulated sugar

1 egg

1 teaspoon vanilla

ingredients: crumb topping

½ cup butter (room temperature)

1 cup brown sugar

1½ cups flour

½ teaspoon salt

½ teaspoon cinnamon

ingredients: glaze

1 cup powdered sugar

3 tablespoons milk

1 teaspoon corn syrup

directions

1. Preheat oven to 350°F and spray 12 large or 24 small muffin tins with nonstick oil or line with cupcake papers.

4. In a small bowl, mix flour, baking powder, salt, cinnamon, and pumpkin pie spice.

3. In a large bowl, cream the butter and sugars together until completely smooth.

4. Add eggs and vanilla. Mix well.

5. Slowly add the flour mixture to the creamed butter and sugar, alternately adding the buttermilk until all of it is added and incorporated.

6. Fold in the carrots and coconut. Set this batter aside.

7. In a medium bowl, use a hand mixer to combine cream cheese and ¼ cup sugar until smooth. Add egg and vanilla and blend on low until no lumps remain.

8. Pour carrot cake batter into the prepared muffin tins, until each tin is three-quarters full.

9. Spoon a small layer of the cream cheese mixture on top of the carrot cake layer. Add 1 tablespoon cream cheese and swirl into batter.

10. In a small bowl, combine the crumb topping ingredients butter, brown sugar, flour, salt, and cinnamon, and blend with a fork until the mix is crumbly. Sprinkle a small amount on top of each muffin.

11. Bake for 45 to 50 min or until a toothpick comes out clean from the muffin.

12. Let the muffins cool completely.

13. In a small bowl, stir powdered sugar, milk, and corn syrup together to make a thin glaze.

14. When the muffins are cooled, drizzle the glaze over each one.

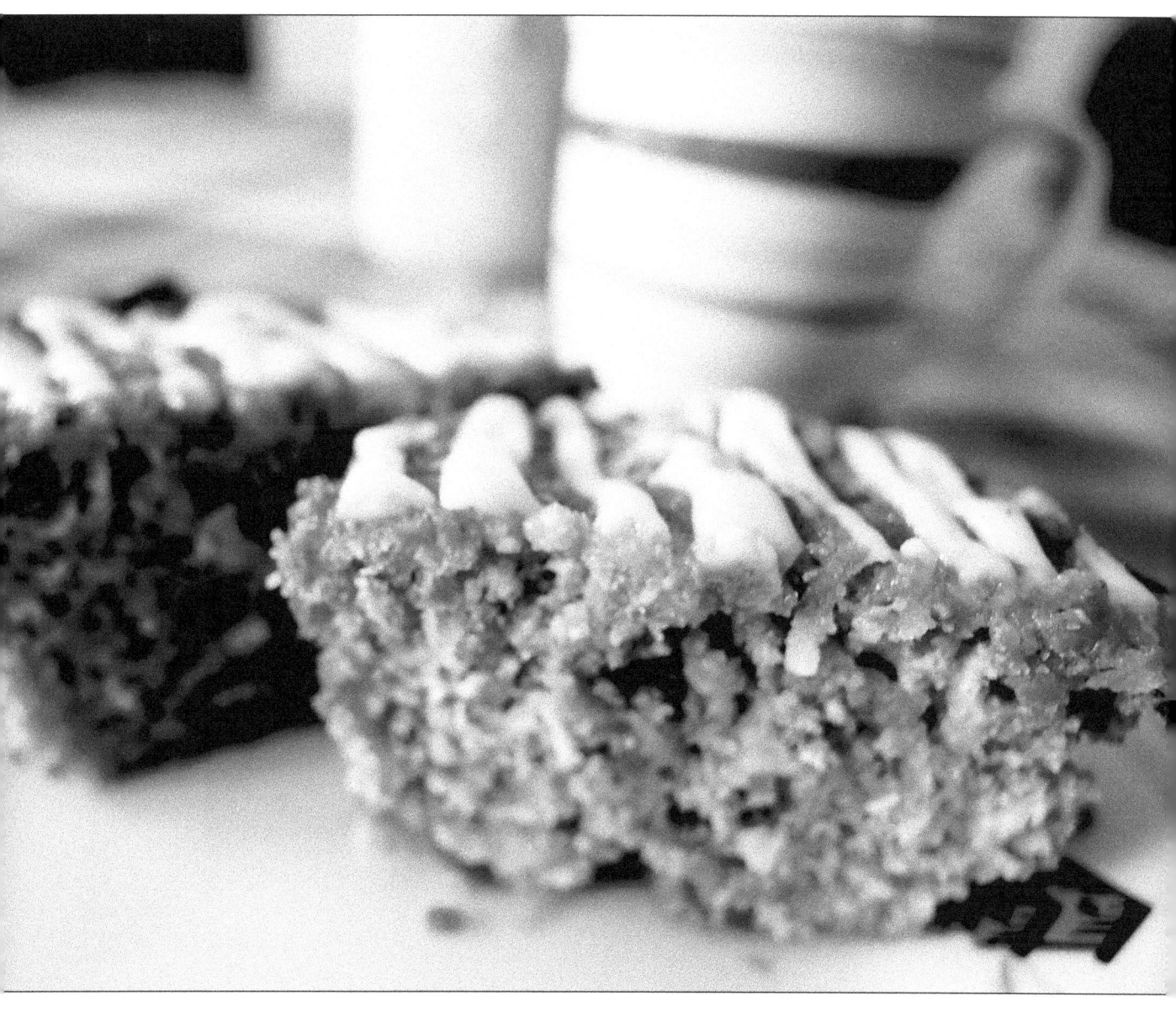

Asparagus Frittata

ingredients

4 ounces chopped prosciutto

8 eggs

½ cup milk

1 teaspoon rosemary

⅛ teaspoon ground black pepper

2 tablespoons olive oil

6 fresh asparagus spears, trimmed and finely minced

½ cup shredded cheddar cheese

Parsley for garnish

directions

1. Preheat oven to 375°F.

2. Place the prosciutto on a parchment-paper-lined cooking sheet. Bake for 10 to 15 minutes. Remove. Set aside to cool.

3. In a medium bowl, whisk eggs, milk, rosemary, and pepper. Set aside.

4. Heat oil over medium heat in a large skillet. Add asparagus and sauté for 1 to 2 minutes. Small pieces will cook quickly.

5. Pour the egg mixture into the skillet over the asparagus.

6. Let it cook, undisturbed, for 1 to 2 minutes, reducing heat if necessary to prevent burning.

7. Using a small spatula, lift the edges of the egg slightly and tilt the skillet, allowing any uncooked egg to run to the bottom.

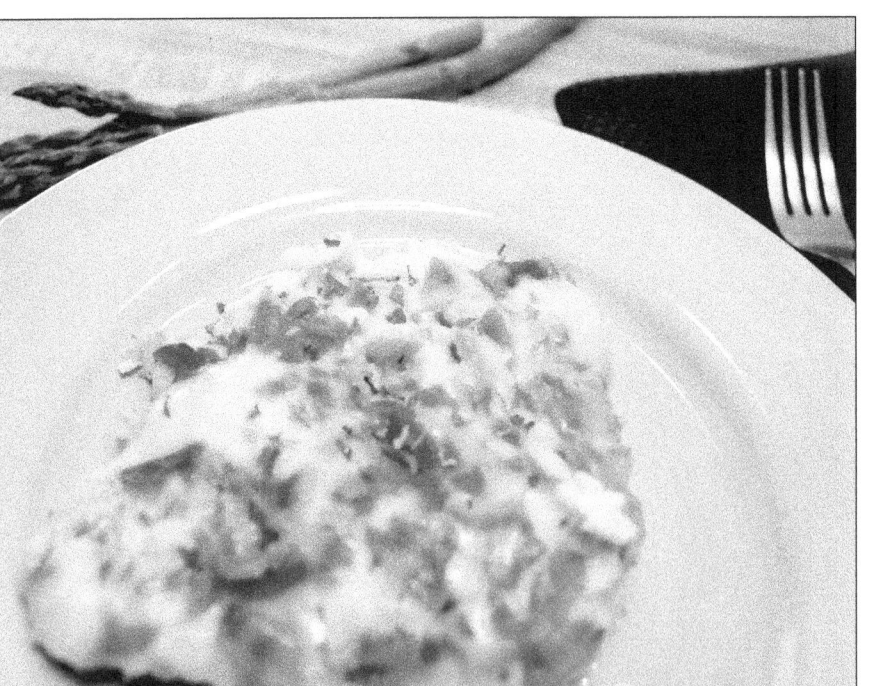

8. Add the chopped prosciutto and cheddar cheese.

9. Reduce heat to low, cover, and cook for 1 minute or until the cheese has melted.

10. Use the spatula to lift away the edges and bottom of the frittata.

11. Tip the pan gently over a serving platter, allowing the frittata to slide onto the platter.

12. Cut into wedges, garnish with parsley if desired, and serve warm.

Sausage and Chard Frittata

directions

1. In a large skillet over medium heat cook the sausage until it is browned and crisp. Transfer to a paper towel-lined plate to remove excess grease. Set aside.

2. In the same skillet, add 1 tablespoon of olive oil, tilting the pan slightly to distribute the oil so it heats evenly. Add leeks and cook for 1 minute or until translucent.

3. Add potatoes, salt, and pepper, then and cook for 5 minutes, stirring occasionally.

4. Add in the cooked sausage or chorizo.

5. In a large bowl, whisk eggs with **Swiss chard purée**, cheese, and herbs.

6. Pour the egg mixture evenly into the skillet, covering the potatoes and sausage.

7. Let the mix cook, undisturbed, for 2 minutes.

8. Using a small spatula, lift the edges of the egg slightly and tilt the skillet, allowing any uncooked egg to run to the bottom.

9. Reduce heat, cover, and cook for an additional 2 minutes, checking frequently to prevent burning.

10. Use the spatula to loosen the edges and bottom of the frittata.

11. Tip the pan gently over a serving platter, allowing the frittata to slide onto the platter.

12. Cut into wedges and serve.

ingredients

- 4 ounces thinly sliced smoked sausage or chorizo
- 1 tablespoon olive oil
- ¼ cup diced leeks
- 2 cups shredded hash browned potatoes
- ½ teaspoon salt
- ½ teaspoon pepper
- 8 eggs
- ½ cup **Swiss chard purée**
- ⅓ cup grated Monterey jack or mozzarella cheese
- 1 teaspoon parsley
- 1 teaspoon rosemary
- 1 teaspoon oregano

Breakfast Turnovers

ingredients

7 eggs (divided)

½ cup **puréed kale**

½ teaspoon kosher salt

¼ teaspoon ground black pepper

1 teaspoon dried thyme leaves

4 sheets puff pastry, thawed

2 tablespoons olive oil

8 ounce sliced ham or cooked and crumbled breakfast meat

1 cup grated Gouda or Gruyere cheese

2 tablespoons water

directions

1. Preheat oven to 400°F. Line a baking sheet with parchment paper.
2. In a large bowl, whisk 6 of the eggs with the **puréed kale,** salt, pepper, and thyme.
3. Pour the whisked egg onto a prepared sheet pan and bake for 15 minutes, or until the egg is cooked through.
4. Remove the egg mixture from the oven and place on a cooling rack for 10 minutes. When cooled, cut into four large squares, then cut each square at an angle to create eight triangles. Set aside.
5. Reset temperature to 375°F.
6. Line a second baking sheet with parchment paper.
7. In a small bowl, create an egg wash by pouring the 2 tablespoons of water into a small bowl and adding the remaining egg. Whisk to blend and set aside.
8. Roll one pastry out on a floured surface into an 11-inch square.
9. Place a layer of ham or other cooked meat on one half of the dough, leaving a 1-inch border of pastry.
10. Add a triangle of cooked egg, topped with cheese.
11. Add a second layer of ham or breakfast meat, another egg triangle, and cheese.
12. Using the egg wash to moisten the 1-inch border of the pastry, fold it over and press lightly to seal the edge.
13. Carefully transfer the pastry to the parchment paper.
14. Repeat steps 8 to 13 with the remaining three pastries.
15. Brush the top of each pastry with the remaining egg wash.
16. Cut 3 vents on top of each. Bake for 10 minutes, then rotate the baking sheet in the oven. Continue baking for an additional 10 minutes, or until the pastry's crust is golden brown and puffed.
17. Cool on a rack for 10 to 15 min. Serve warm or at room temperature.

Nutty Egg Waffles

directions

1. Preheat a waffle iron.

2. In a medium-sized bowl, whisk eggs, minced Brussels sprouts, nutmeg, walnuts, salt, and pepper, then set aside.

3. Lightly grease the waffle maker with cooking spray.

4. Pour ¼ of the egg mixture into the waffle maker, sprinkle ham, and top with cheese. Do not overfill.

5. Close the waffle iron and cook until it's done and golden brown; that is, for about 3 minutes.

6. The waffles will be crunchy with a nutty flavor and will pair well with honey mustard for a savory treat or maple syrup for a sweet one.

ingredients

8 eggs

1 cup minced Brussels sprouts

½ teaspoon nutmeg

¼ teaspoon ground walnuts

½ teaspoon salt

¼ teaspoon freshly ground black pepper

1 ½ cups grated cheddar cheese

1 cup finely diced ham

Honey mustard for topping (optional)

cooking spray

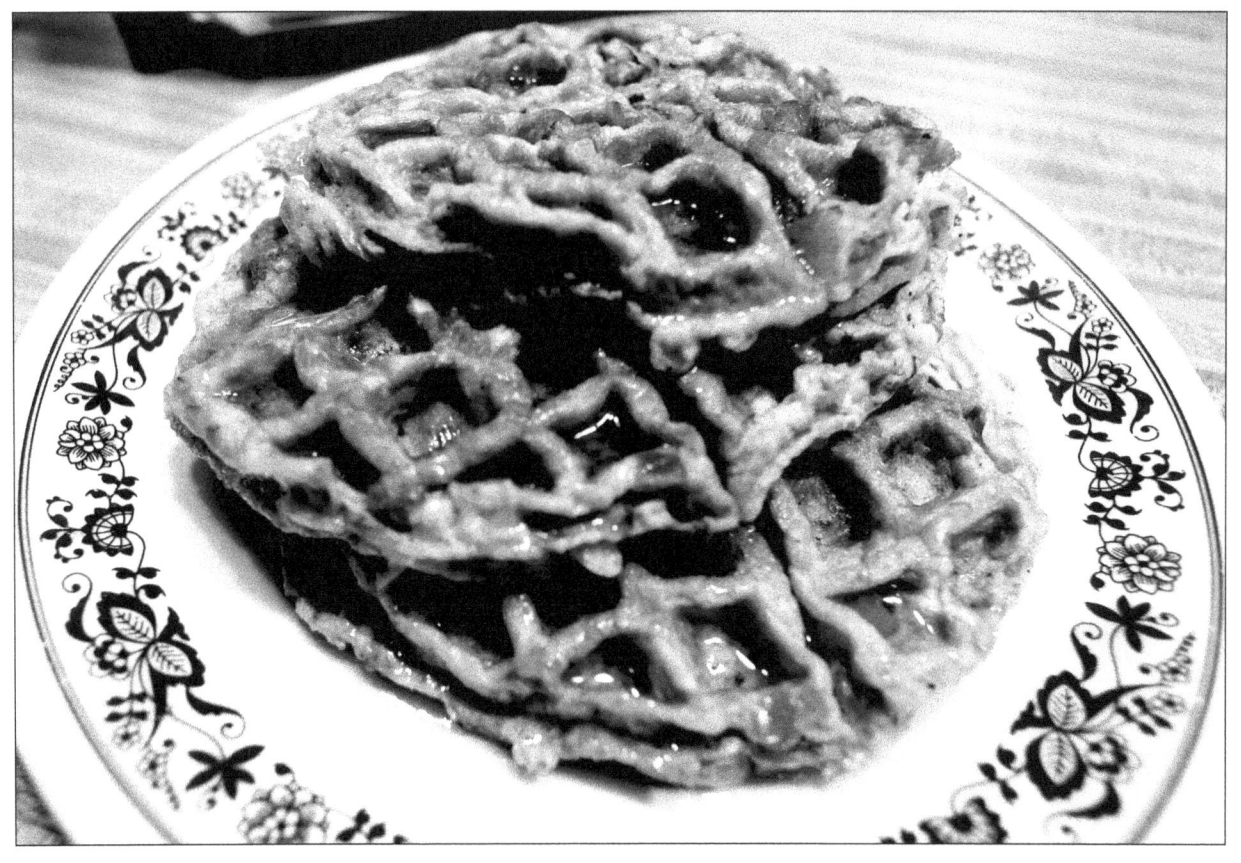

Morning Potato Nachos

ingredients

1 tablespoon olive oil

1 teaspoon salt

½ teaspoon ground cumin

¼ teaspoon ground chipotle pepper

2 whole sweet potatoes, peeled

5 slices bacon

4 eggs

½ teaspoon olive oil

¼ teaspoon pepper

¼ teaspoon salt

1 diced jalapeño, seeds removed (optional)

Smooth Salsa (recipe page 61)

½ cup shredded cheddar cheese

directions

1. Preheat oven to 400°F.

2. Line a baking sheet with parchment paper.

3. Pour the olive oil into a large bowl. Set aside.

4. In a medium bowl, whisk the salt, cumin, and chipotle. Set aside.

5. Slice the sweet potatoes into ¼ inch rounds.

6. Add all the rounds to the olive oil and toss to coat.

7. Transfer the sweet potato rounds to the bowl with the spices and toss to completely cover.

8. Spread in a single layer on the parchment paper on the sheet.

9. Bake for 15 minutes.

10. Remove from oven and use tongs to flip the rounds over. Return the sheet to the oven and bake for another 15 minutes.

11. While the potatoes are baking, prepare the toppings.

12. Cook the bacon in a skillet over medium heat for 2 to 3 minutes until it reaches the desired doneness. Remove from heat and set on a paper towel to drain fat. When cooled, chop into small sections.

13. Whisk the eggs with olive oil, salt, and pepper. Add diced jalapeño if using.

14. Pour into the skillet and scramble.

15. Remove the sweet potato rounds from the oven and transfer to a serving dish. Sprinkle ¼ cup of cheddar cheese.

16. Top the rounds with eggs and chopped bacon, drizzle with smooth salsa, and sprinkle with the remaining cheddar cheese.

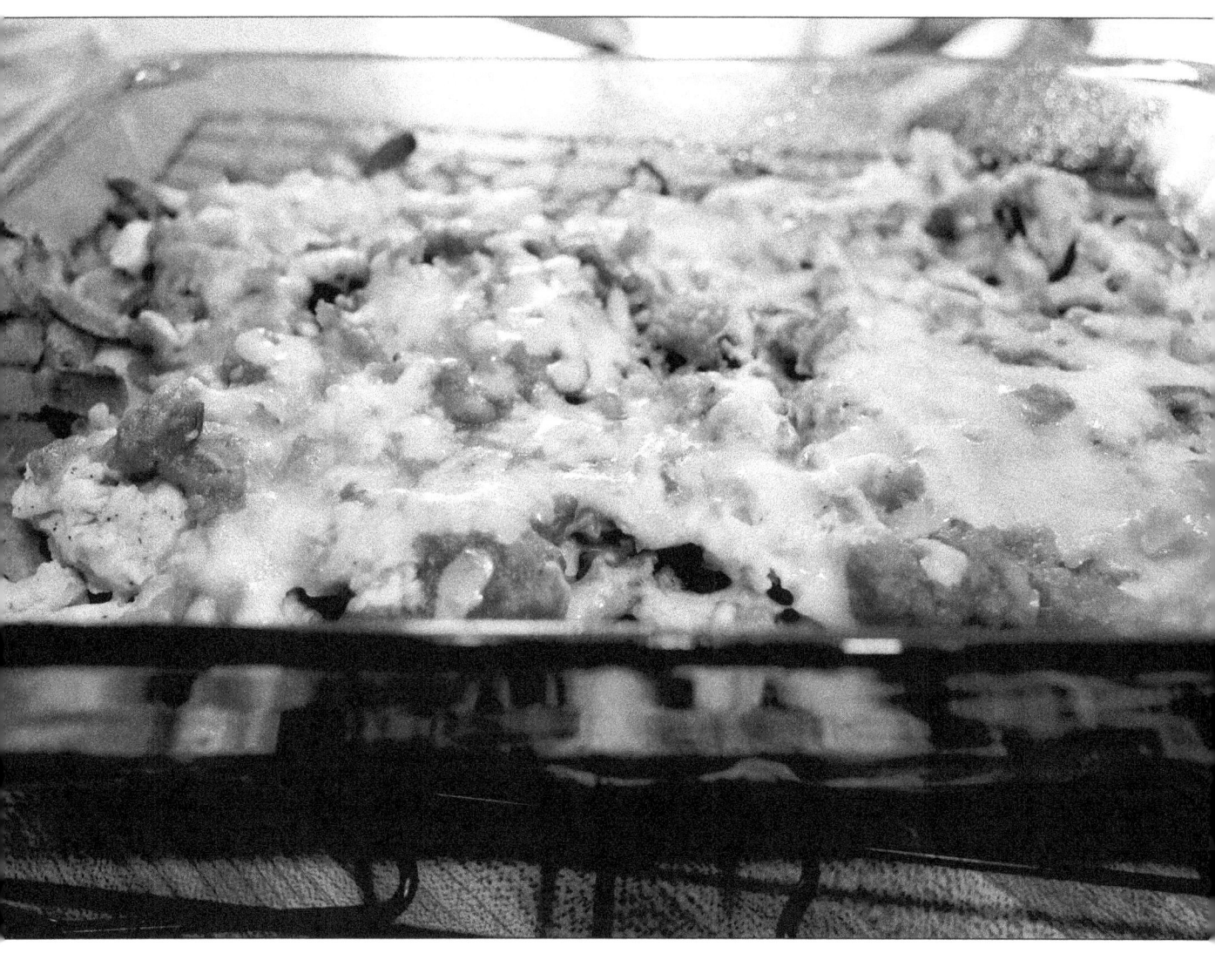

Bacon and Cheese Quiche

ingredients

One 9-inch deep dish frozen pie crust

1 teaspoon olive oil

4 strips of bacon

¼ cup **minced leeks**

½ cup **spinach purée**

5 ounces shredded Gruyere or Havarti cheese

3 ounces grated Parmesan cheese

4 eggs

¼ teaspoon salt

¼ teaspoon pepper

1 cup half-and-half

directions

1. Preheat the oven to 400° F.

2. Place uncooked pie crust in a pie pan on a baking sheet.

3. Pour olive oil into a skillet over medium heat. Add bacon and cook until the bacon is very well done but not burnt. Remove and set on a paper towel to cool.

4. Using the skillet with bacon grease, add **leeks** and cook over medium heat for 5 to 8 minutes until they are translucent.

5. In a medium bowl, mix the leeks, cheese, and **spinach.** Add crumbled bacon. Mix well.

6. Spread on pie crust in a smooth layer.

7. In a small bowl, whisk eggs with salt, pepper, and half-and-half until blended.

8. Pour the egg mixture over the cheese and spinach mixture.

9. Bake for 15 minutes.

10. Reduce heat to 350° F and bake for an additional 30 to 35 minutes or until the top of the quiche begins to turn golden brown.

Crockpot Breakfast Casserole

directions

1. Cook the sausage with **leeks** and **peppers** in a large skillet over medium heat until browned and crumbled. Drain fat and set aside.

2. In the same skillet, cook bacon to the desired doneness, remove, and set on paper towels to drain fat.

3. In a large bowl, whisk together **puréed kale,** eggs, milk, salt, pepper, and sour cream.

4. Spray the inside of a 6-quart slow cooker with cooking spray.

5. Place half the frozen hash browns in the bottom of the slow cooker.

6. Add a layer of half the sausage. Crumble the bacon and add half of it over the sausage.

7. Sprinkle 1 cup of shredded cheese.

8. Spread the remaining frozen hash browns as the next layer.

9. Add the remaining sausage and bacon.

10. Pour the egg and kale mixture evenly over the top.

11. Cover and cook on low for 6 to 8 hours or for 2 to 3 hours on high.

12. Before serving, add the remaining cheese and replace the cover for 5 to 10 minutes to allow the cheese to melt.

ingredients

½ lb of breakfast sausage

1 cup minced leeks

1 cup **diced bell pepper**

½ lb of bacon

A 1-lb package of frozen shredded hash brown potatoes

2 cups shredded cheddar cheese, divided

1 cup **puréed kale**

12 eggs

¾ cup milk

½ cup sour cream

½ teaspoon salt

¼ teaspoon ground black pepper

Glazed Beet Donuts

ingredients

2⅓ cups all-purpose flour

2½ teaspoons baking powder

1½ teaspoons ground cinnamon

1 teaspoon nutmeg

1 teaspoon grated orange peel

¼ teaspoon salt

1 egg

¼ cup **beet juice**

⅓ cup packed light brown sugar

1 cup buttermilk

⅓ cup sour cream

2½ teaspoons vanilla extract

ingredients: glaze

1 cup powdered sugar

1 teaspoon vanilla

1–2 tablespoons of milk, depending on desired thickness

Sprinkles (optional)

directions

1. Preheat the oven to 350°F.

2. Spray a donut pan with non-stick spray. Set aside.

3. In a large bowl, whisk the flour, baking powder, cinnamon, nutmeg, grated orange peel, and salt. Set aside.

4. Blend the egg, **beet juice,** brown sugar, buttermilk, sour cream, and vanilla extract in a medium bowl until smooth.

5. Pour the wet ingredients into the dry ingredients and mix until just combined. Do not overmix.

6. Spoon the batter into the donut cavities up to about ¾ full.

7. Bake for 10 to 11 minutes or until the top is firm and a toothpick comes out clean.

8. Allow to cool for about two minutes and transfer to a wire rack set on a large piece of parchment paper or on a baking sheet (for easier cleanup).

9. To prepare the glaze: In a medium bowl, mix powdered sugar, vanilla, and milk until smooth. Less milk will result in a heavier glaze, while more milk will create a thinner icing.

10. Hold each donut by the edges and dip the top into the glaze.

11. Place the glazed donuts on a wire rack to let the glaze set for 3 to 4 minutes. Dip a second time if desired. If using, add sprinkles after the second dip.

12. Donuts are best served immediately. Store leftovers loosely covered at room temperature for up to 2 days, or freeze.

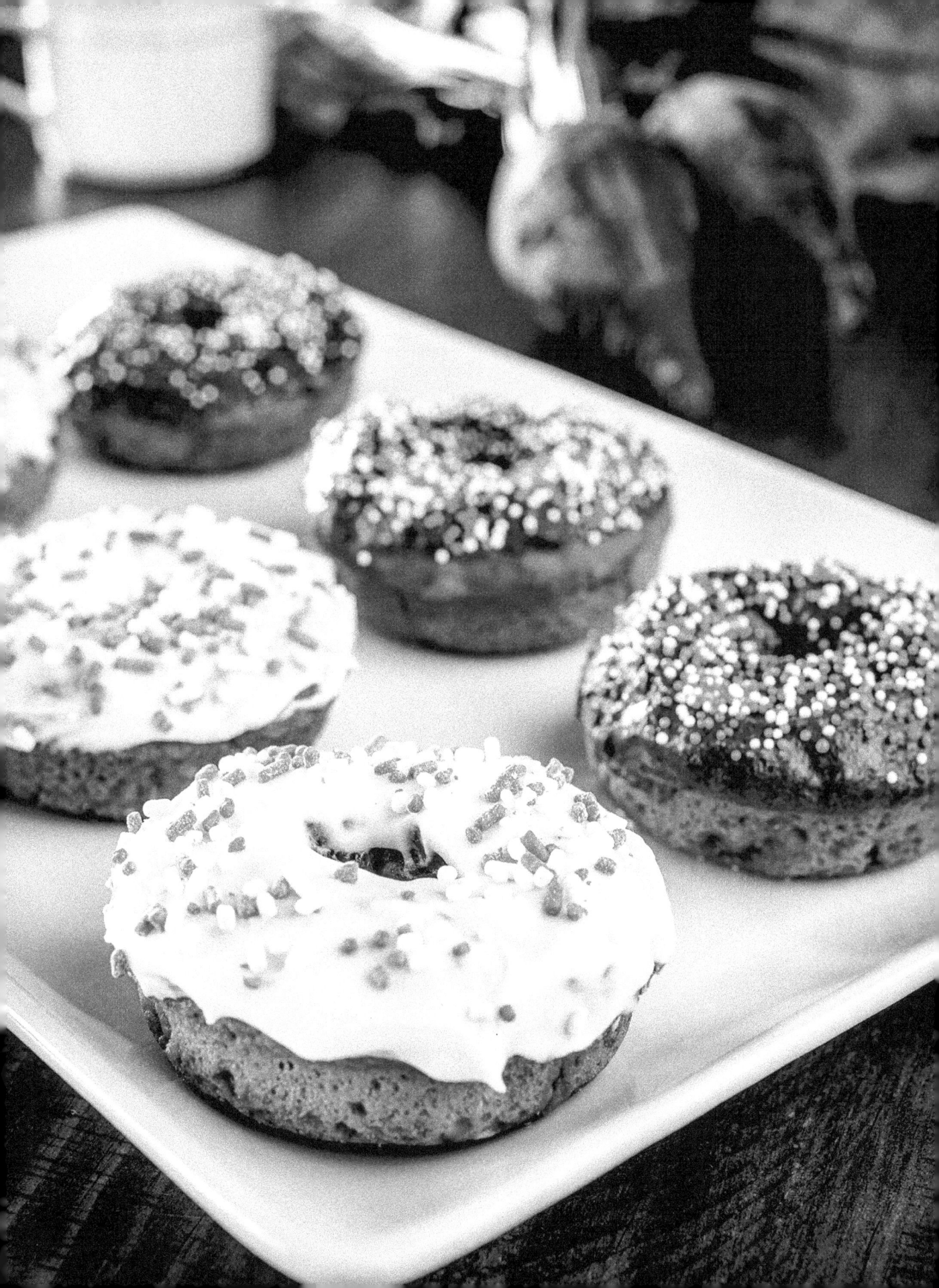

Banana Cauliflower Muffins

ingredients

⅓ cup unsalted butter

3 large ripe bananas, mashed

¾ cup sugar

1 egg

1 teaspoon baking powder

1 teaspoon baking soda

½ teaspoon salt

½ teaspoon ginger

½ cup riced cauliflower

1½ cups flour

Walnuts or pecans

directions

1. Preheat oven to 375°F.
2. Melt the butter in the microwave then set aside to cool.
3. Spray muffin tin with non-stick spray. Set aside.
4. In a large bowl, mash bananas with a fork or pastry cutter.
5. Add sugar, egg, and melted butter.
6. In a separate bowl, whisk the flour, baking powder, baking soda, ginger, and salt.
7. Add to the batter and stir until just combined.
8. Fold in riced cauliflower and nuts.
9. Spoon the batter into the prepared muffin tin.
10. Bake for 20 minutes.
11. Remove the muffins from the pan immediately; place on a wire rack to cool.

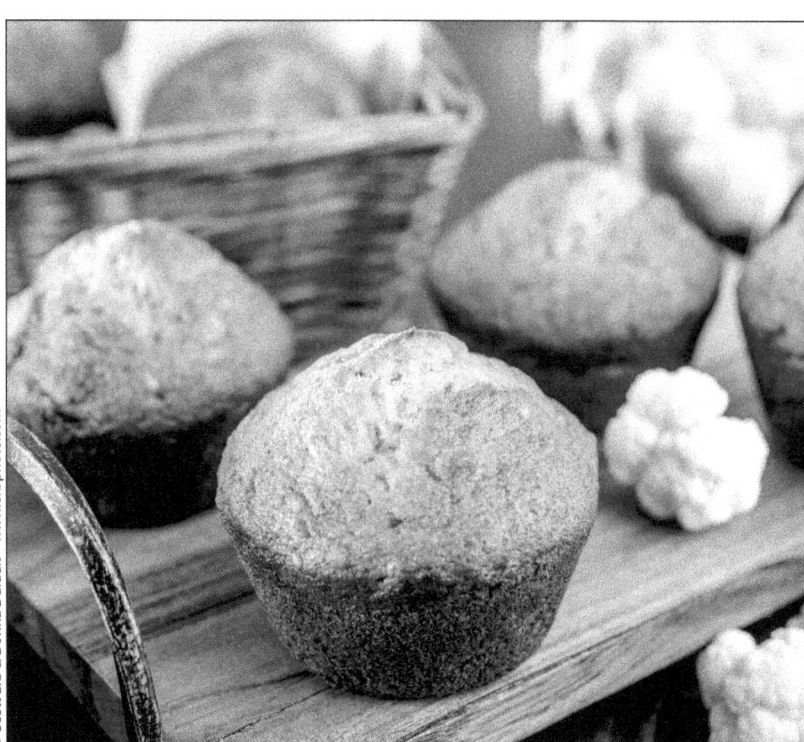

Pumpkin-Cranberry Muffins

directions

1. Preheat oven to 375°F.
2. Spray muffin tin with non-stick spray. Set aside.
3. In a large bowl, combine sugar, brown sugar, pumpkin, buttermilk, canola oil, and egg. Mix well.
4. In a medium bowl, whisk together flour, baking soda, ginger, baking powder, cinnamon, salt, and cloves.
5. Add the flour mixture to the sugar mixture and stir until just combined.
6. Fold in the cranberries.
7. Spoon the batter into the prepared muffin tin.
8. Bake for 25 minutes or until the muffins spring back when touched lightly in the center.
9. Remove the muffins from the pan immediately; place on a wire rack to cool.

ingredients

1 cup granulated sugar

¼ cup packed light brown sugar

1 cup pumpkin purée

½ cup buttermilk

2 tablespoons canola oil

1 egg

1½ cups all-purpose flour

1 teaspoon baking soda

¾ teaspoon ground ginger

½ teaspoon baking powder

½ teaspoon ground cinnamon

¼ teaspoon salt

⅛ teaspoon ground cloves

½ cup whole cranberries

Omelet Muffins

ingredients

1 lb seasoned breakfast sausage

1 cup **minced red bell pepper**

1 cup minced leeks

8 eggs

¼ teaspoon salt

⅛ teaspoon ground black pepper

2 tablespoons water

4 ounce shredded cheddar cheese

directions

1. Preheat oven to 350°F.

2. Spray muffin tins with nonstick oil or use paper liners.

3. Cook the sausage in a large skillet over medium heat until browned and crumbled. Drain fat and set aside.

4. In a large bowl, whisk together eggs, salt, black pepper, and water.

5. Add the cooked sausage, **minced bell pepper,** and minced leeks. Stir to combine.

6. Pour the mixture evenly into prepared muffin cups.

7. Top each with cheddar cheese.

8. Bake for 18 to 20 minutes or until the muffins are set in the middle.

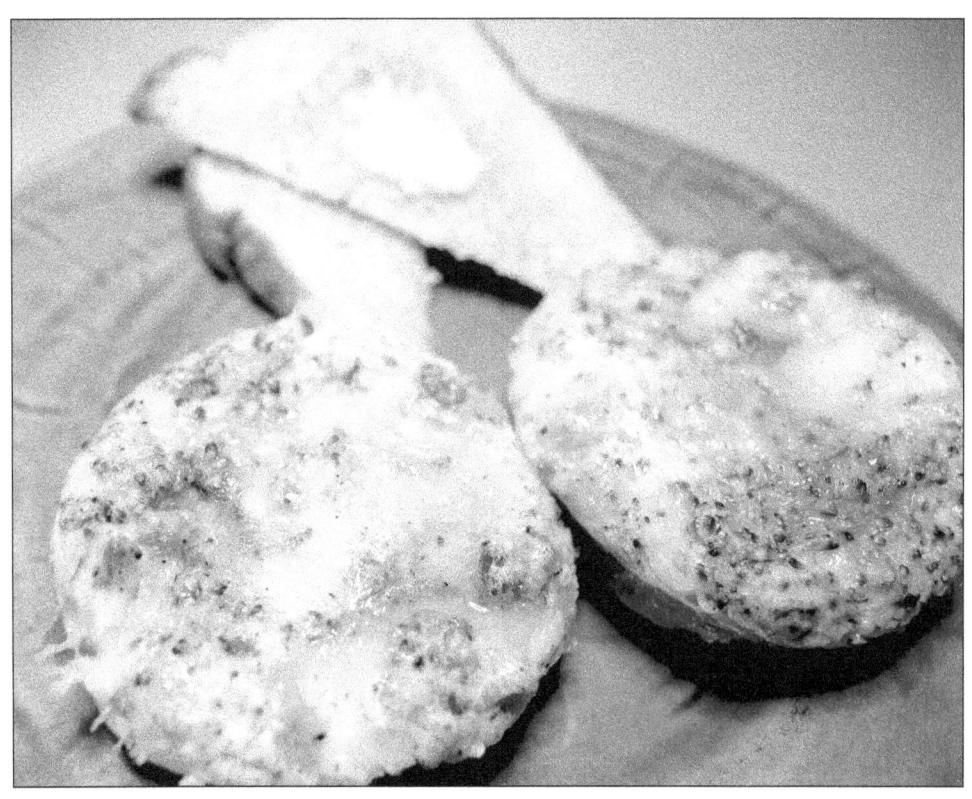

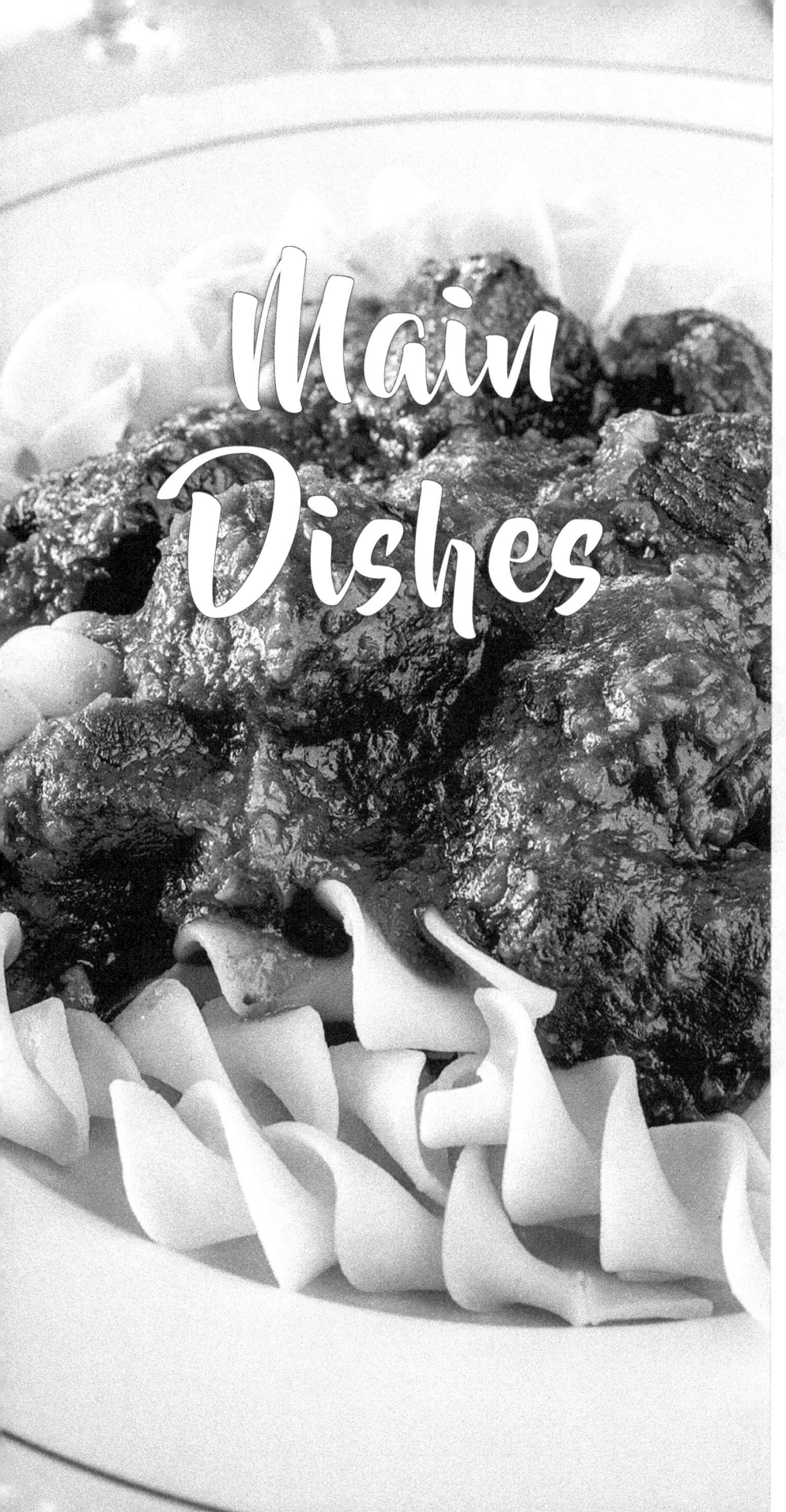

Main Dishes

- 108 Beef Bourguignon
- 110 Chicken Enchiladas
- 112 Beef Po Boys on Spinach Bun
- 112 Cornbread Meatloaf
- 113 Too Good to Be Veggie Lasagna
- 114 Spinach Salisbury Steak
- 116 Cheeseburger Pockets
- 117 Beef Hotpot
- 118 Fresh Veggie Noodles
- 120 Homemade Chicken Pot Pie
- 121 Pumpkin Beef Stew
- 122 Veggie Peanut Chicken and Zucchini Noodles
- 124 Shepherd's Pie
- 125 Pepperoni Spinach Roll-Up
- 126 Chicken Tetrazzini with Asparagus
- 128 Skillet Ziti with Sausage & Kale
- 129 Stuffed Pasta Shells
- 130 Sloppy Joes
- 131 Crock Pot Pasta Bolognese-style Sauce
- 132 Western Beef and Corn Casserole
- 133 Sausage & Kohlrabi Fettuccini

Beef Bourguignon

ingredients

1 tablespoon olive oil

3 lbs chuck steak or stewing meat cut into 2-inch chunks

½ cup riced carrots

¾ cup minced onion (about 1 large)

6 garlic cloves, minced

¼ teaspoon salt

¼ teaspoon pepper

2 tablespoons flour

3 cups red wine

1 teaspoon thyme

2 tablespoons parsley

2 bay leaves

⅓ cup **beet purée**

2 cups beef stock

1 tablespoon tomato paste

1 beef bouillon cube, crushed

2 tablespoons butter

directions

1. In a large Dutch oven or stockpot, add olive oil and warm for 1 minute over medium heat. Add beef and sear until it is browned on all sides. Remove the beef and set aside.

2. Sauté the carrots and minced onions with the minced garlic for 1 minute in the remaining oil.

3. Add the beef back to the pot.

4. Mix salt and pepper with the flour and add to the pot, tossing to coat the beef. Cook for 4 to 5 minutes to brown.

5. Add the wine and herbs.

6. In a medium bowl, mix the **beet purée,** beef stock, and tomato paste, whisking to blend, then add to the stockpot.

7. Bring to a simmer on the stove.

8. Cover and simmer on low heat for 2 to 3 hours, or until the meat is tender and falls apart.

9. Do not cook down the liquid. About 2½ cups of sauce should remain with the meat when done.

10. Serve with mashed potatoes, rice, or noodles.

More Hidden Veggies! Serve over Mashed Rutabaga or Sweet Potatoes.

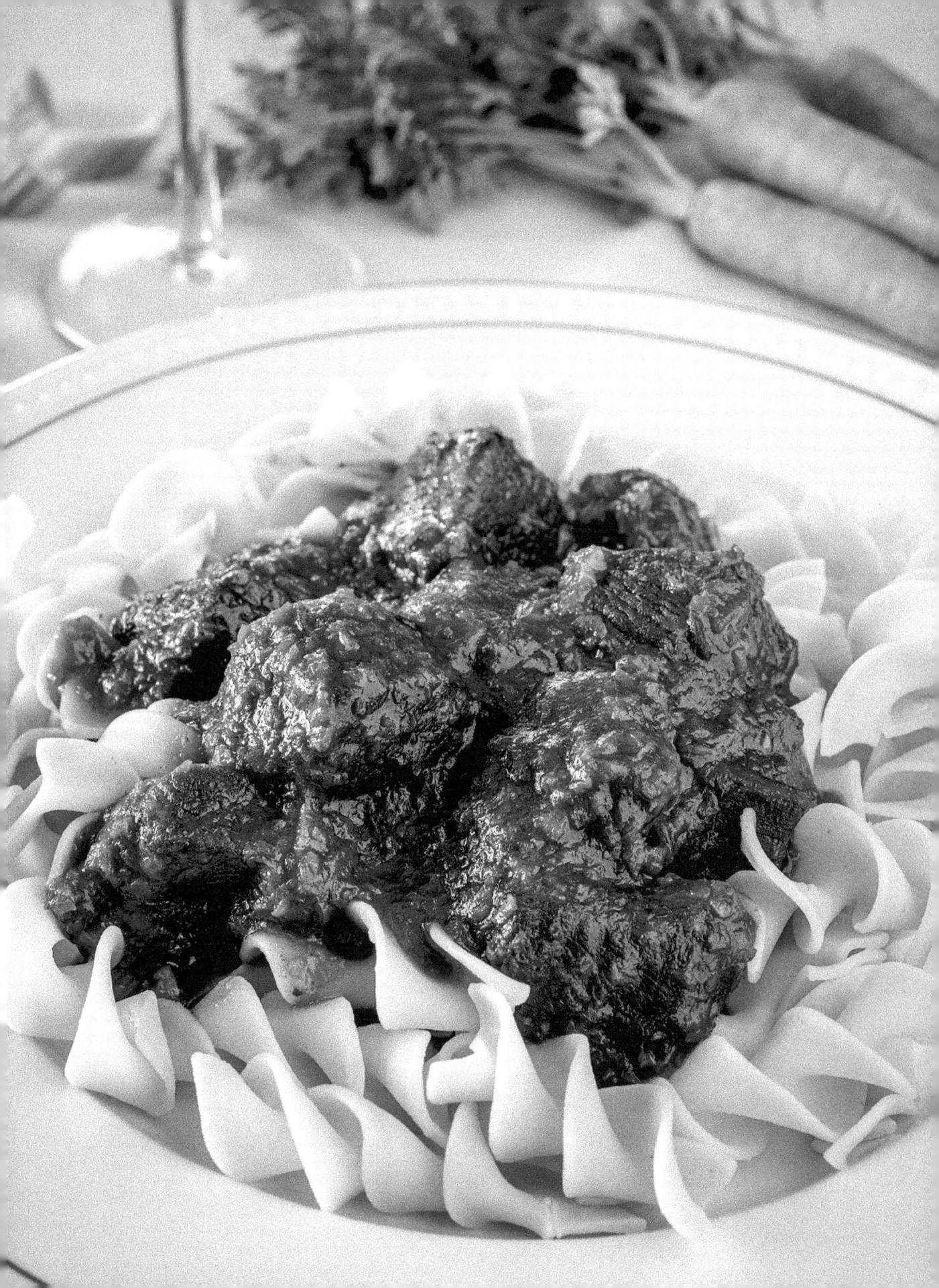

Chicken Enchiladas

ingredients

4 cups cold water

2 cups chicken broth

1 celery stalk, chopped into 3 large pieces

2 carrots, peeled and chopped into 2-inch pieces

1 jalapeño pepper, cut in half with seeds removed

½ medium onion, cut into large wedges

1 tablespoon fresh ground pepper

5 cloves of garlic, chopped

12 ounce boneless chicken breast, cut in quarters

1 cup green enchilada sauce

½ cup fresh diced tomatoes or a 14.5 ounce can diced tomatoes

4 oz. cream cheese

1 teaspoon dried cilantro

½ teaspoon ground cumin

¼ teaspoon salt

¼ teaspoon ground red pepper

Twelve 6-inch corn tortillas

Cooking spray

½ cup shredded Mexican blend cheese

directions

1. In a large saucepan, combine the water, chicken broth, and pepper, stirring to mix. Add celery, carrot, jalapeno, onion, and garlic. Add chicken and place over medium heat. Bring to a simmer and cook for 10 to 12 minutes until the chicken is done.

2. Remove chicken and set aside.

3. While the chicken is cooling, use a colander set over a large bowl or pot to strain the liquid from the onions, carrots, celery, and jalapeños.

4. Put the strained liquid back into the saucepan, place on the stove, and add the enchilada sauce.

5. Spoon all the vegetables from the colander into a food processor and blend until puréed (*see* Note next page). Add 1 to 2 tablespoons of the liquid from the saucepan into the food processor if needed to achieve a smooth purée.

6. Pour half the purée into a medium-sized bowl and the remaining amount back into the saucepan on the stove with the enchilada sauce.

7. Bring to a boil then reduce heat and simmer until the liquid is reduced to about 2 cups. This may take 30–40 minutes.

8. While the sauce is simmering, shred the chicken using two forks or a food processor. Add the chicken to the medium-sized bowl with the puréed vegetables.

9. Add tomatoes, cream cheese, cilantro, cumin, salt, and red pepper. Stir to mix well. Cover and refrigerate while the sauce is simmering.

10. When the simmering liquid is reduced, remove from heat.

11. Preheat the oven to 400°F.

12. Prepare an 11x7 baking dish with cooking spray. Cover the bottom with ¼ cup of the cooked enchilada sauce.

Chicken Enchiladas (continued)

13. Remove the shredded chicken mixture from the refrigerator.

14. Warm each tortilla in a skillet at low heat for 10 to 15 seconds per side or until soft. Lay flat and fill with about ⅓ cup of the shredded chicken mixture; roll up. Place seam side down in the prepared baking dish.

15. When all the chicken has been used, pour the simmered sauce over the enchiladas.

16. Top with cheddar cheese.

17. Bake at 400°F for 20 minutes or until lightly browned.

18. Serve warm.

NOTE: If the sauce is too spicy, do not add jalapeño to the purée mix. Or, take ½ cup purée mix and add back into the food processor with the jalapeno. Reserve in a side dish to serve as a topping for those who like a hotter flavor.

TIP: Cooking the chicken with whole vegetables helps add the flavor!

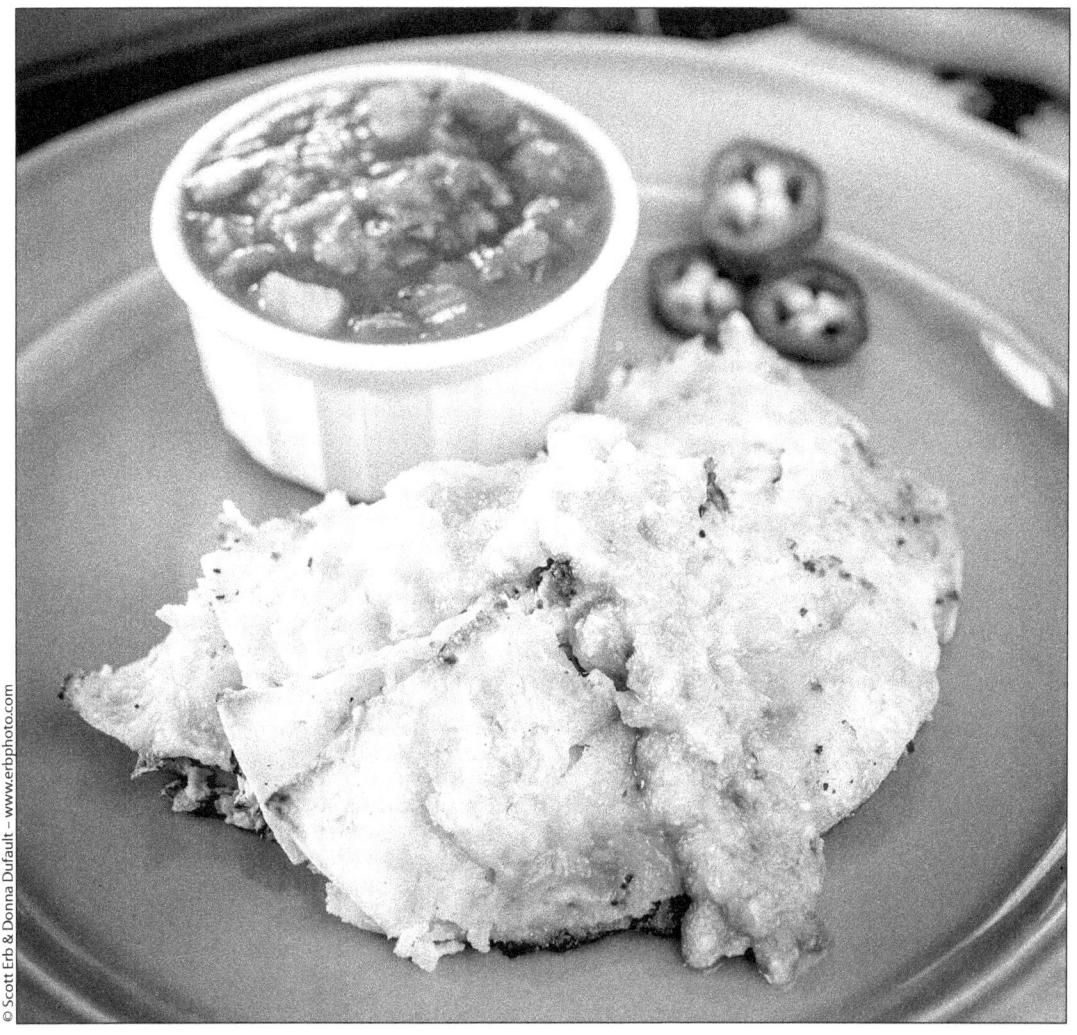

Beef Po Boys on Spinach Bun

ingredients

2–3 lbs of boneless beef roast

¼ cup dry red wine

3 tablespoons apple cider vinegar

1 cup beef bouillon

1 tablespoon Worcestershire sauce

½ teaspoon garlic powder

½ teaspoon dried thyme

½ teaspoon basil

1 cup minced leeks or onion

2 cups riced carrots

Spinach Burger Buns (p. 80)

directions

1. Place the beef roast in a slow cooker.

2. In a medium bowl, combine the red wine, apple cider vinegar, beef bouillon, Worcestershire, thyme, basil, and garlic powder. Whisk until blended.

3. Pour this mixture over the roast in a slow cooker, then add leeks or onion and carrots.

4. Cover and cook on low for 8 to 10 hours, or until the beef is very tender.

5. Remove the beef from the slow cooker and cool slightly before shredding.

6. Pour sauce into individual serving bowls for dipping sauce.

7. Spoon beef into the spinach buns and serve with sauce.

Cornbread Meatloaf

ingredients

2 lbs of lean ground beef

1 egg

¼ cup ketchup

1 tablespoon Worcestershire sauce

1 packet of cornbread stuffing

1 teaspoon garlic powder

1 teaspoon seasoning salt

½ teaspoon pepper

½ cup minced leeks or onions

½ cup riced carrots

¼ cup minced celery

2 tablespoons barbeque sauce

directions

1. Preheat oven to 350°F.

2. Add all ingredients to a large bowl.

3. Mix with a spoon or hands until thoroughly combined.

4. Place in a 9x5 bread loaf pan, pressing down firmly.

5. Spread the barbeque sauce on top of the mixture.

6. Bake for 60 minutes.

7. Serve immediately.

Too Good to Be Veggie Lasagna

directions

1. Preheat oven to 375°F.
2. Brown the ground beef and Italian sausage in a skillet over medium heat until completely cooked and no pink remains. Drain excess fat.
3. Return to heat. Stir in diced carrots and red pepper flakes. Cook for 2 to 3 minutes more.
4. Remove from heat. Set aside to cool.
5. Prepare lasagna noodles according to package directions.
6. In a large bowl, mix the two jars of sauce with the **spinach purée.**
7. In a second bowl, mix the Ricotta cheese and mozzarella cheese.
8. When the pasta is ready, drain in a colander and run under cool water until you can comfortably touch it with your hands.
9. In a 9x13 pan at least 3 inches deep, pour ¼ cup sauce over the bottom.
10. Place a layer of noodles side by side in the sauce, covering the entire surface of the pan.
11. Pour another ½ cup of sauce on top of the noodles. Spread ⅓ of the meat, followed by ⅓ of the Ricotta/mozzarella cheese blend, then ⅓ of the cheddar cheese. Top with another layer of noodles.
12. Repeat the sauce, meat, and cheese layers.
13. Continue until all the ingredients are consumed.
14. Bake for 60 to 75 minutes or until lightly browned and bubbly.
15. Remove from oven. Allow to set for at least 15 minutes before cutting.

ingredients

1 lb ground beef

1 lb spicy Italian sausage

½ cup minced carrots

1 teaspoon crushed red pepper flakes

One 16-ounce packet of lasagna noodles

Two 24-ounce jars of pasta sauce (garlic, spicy, or flavored with meat)

¾ cup **spinach purée**

One 15-ounce can of Ricotta cheese

16 ounce shredded mozzarella

16 ounce sharp cheddar or cheddar-jack blend

Spinach Salisbury Steak

ingredients: steaks

2 lbs of ground beef

1 egg

½ cup breadcrumbs

1 teaspoon granulated garlic

1 tablespoon ketchup

2 teaspoons dried mustard

1 teaspoon Worcestershire sauce

1 cube crumbled beef bouillon

1 tablespoon hickory vinegar or other seasoning sauce

1 teaspoon salt

1 teaspoon black pepper

1 tablespoon olive oil

1 tablespoon butter

ingredients: gravy

1 cup minced onion

2 cups beef broth

3 tablespoons cornstarch

1 cup puréed spinach

1 tablespoon Worcestershire sauce

1 tablespoon ketchup

2 tablespoons hickory vinegar or other seasoning sauce

1 garlic clove, diced

directions

1. In a large bowl, combine the ground beef, egg, breadcrumbs, granulated garlic, ketchup, dry mustard, Worcestershire sauce, crumbled beef bouillon, seasoning sauce, salt, and pepper.

2. Mix by hand until all ingredients are combined well. Form into 6 to 8 oval patties.

3. Fry the patties in a skillet with the butter and oil over medium-high heat, flipping them over until they are no longer pink in the middle.

4. Remove and set aside the patties while you prepare the gravy.

5. Drain excess oil and add **onions** to the skillet. Sauté over medium heat until translucent.

6. Whisk the beef broth and cornstarch in a small bowl. Add **puréed spinach,** Worcestershire sauce, ketchup, vinegar, and garlic. Stir to mix.

7. Add to the skillet with the onions and simmer for 5 to 10 minutes.

8. Add the Salisbury steak patties back into the pan and cover with the gravy. Simmer for 10 minutes more.

9. Serve hot with mashed potatoes or rice.

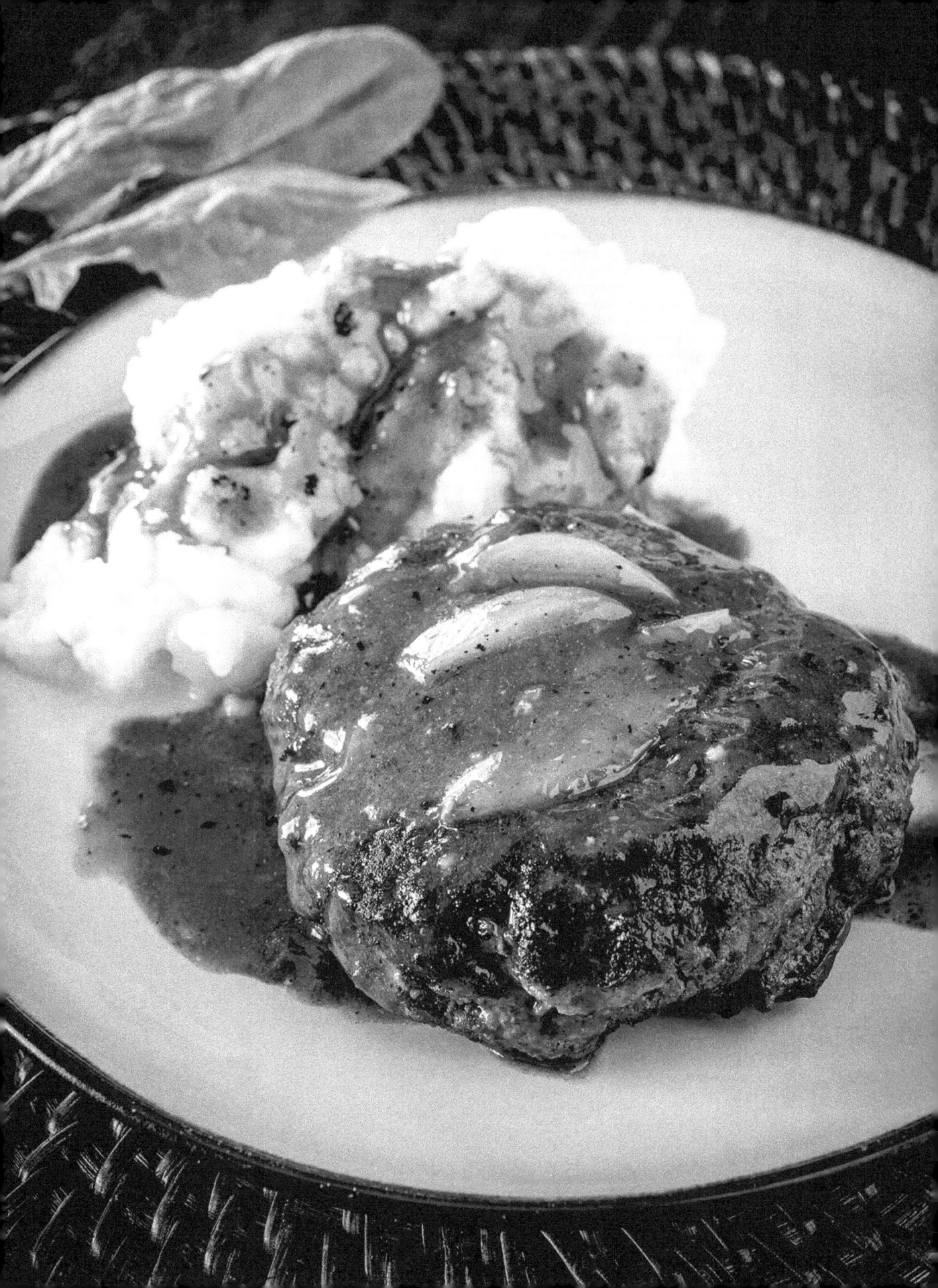

Cheeseburger Pockets

ingredients

1 lb of ground beef

¼ cup chopped leeks or onion

½ cup kale purée

4 tablespoons ketchup

2 tablespoons spicy mustard

½ teaspoon salt

½ teaspoon pepper

Two packages 8-count refrigerated buttermilk biscuits

10 ounces shredded cheddar cheese

1 egg white

1 tablespoon water

4 teaspoons poppy seeds or everything bagel seasoning

directions

1. Preheat oven to 400°F. In a large skillet, cook beef, leeks/onion, salt, and pepper over medium heat until the meat is no longer pink.

2. Drain any fat, then return to medium heat. Stir in kale, ketchup, and mustard. Stir to blend and cook for 1 to 2 minutes.

3. Remove from heat.

4. In a small bowl, whisk together egg white and water to make an egg wash. Set aside.

5. Place two biscuits overlapping on a floured surface; roll out into a 5-inch oval.

6. Place about ¼ cup of the meat mixture on one side and top with cheddar cheese.

7. Fold dough over filling; press edges with a fork to seal.

8. Place on a greased baking sheet.

9. Repeat with the remaining biscuits, meat mixture, and cheese.

10. Prick the top of each lightly with a fork to allow steam to release when baking.

11. Bake for 10 minutes or until golden brown.

12. Remove from oven, brush with egg wash, then top with poppy seeds or everything bagel seasoning.

13. Return to oven for 3 to 5 minutes more.

14. Serve immediately.

Beef Hotpot

directions

1. Preheat oven to 350°F.
2. Warm the olive oil in a large saucepan over medium heat. Add the **leeks** or **onions** and sauté until tender.
3. Add the ground beef and cook until browned. Drain fat.
4. Return the saucepan to heat. Add the **kohlrabi, carrots, Brussels sprouts,** and **peas.**
5. Cook for 3 to 4 minutes, until the vegetables are softened, stirring often to prevent burning.
6. Add flour and stir until blended.
7. Stir in the beef stock, Worcestershire sauce, and horseradish.
8. Bring to a boil.
9. Reduce heat and simmer for 5 minutes.
10. Remove from heat. Spoon into a 9-inch-square baking dish.
11. Lay potato slices on top, overlapping slightly, and brush with melted butter.
12. Cover and bake for 45 minutes.
13. Uncover and continue baking for 10 to 15 minutes more, until the potatoes are brown.
14. Serve immediately.

ingredients

3 tablespoons olive oil

2 cups **diced leeks** or **onions**

1 lb of ground beef

1 teaspoon salt

1 teaspoon pepper

½ cup **minced kohlrabi**

2 cups **riced carrots**

½ cup **riced Brussels sprouts**

1 cup **diced peas**

2 tablespoons flour

2 cups beef stock

4 shakes of Worcestershire Sauce

1 tablespoon horseradish sauce

2–3 medium potatoes, peeled and thinly sliced

3 tablespoons melted butter

Fresh Veggie Noodles

ingredients

2 cups semolina flour or "00" flour

2 eggs

¼ cup **beet, spinach,** carrot, or **kale juice**

1½ tablespoons olive oil

Makes approximately 1 pound

directions

1. Measure out the flour in a large bowl. Using your fingers, create a depression or "well" in the center of the flour pile, just like the crater of a volcano.

2. Slowly pour the **vegetable juice,** eggs, and olive oil into this well.

3. Use a fork to gently blend the liquids, slowly incorporating the flour with the liquid.

4. When it starts making a shaggy dough, start using your hands to blend. When all the flour is incorporated, cover with foil or plastic wrap and allow to sit for 10 minutes.

5. Transfer to a clean, flat surface like a counter, or use a pie mat on a table. Begin kneading by pushing the heel of your hand into the ball of dough, pushing it away from you. Lift half the dough and fold it. Move it one-quarter turn, then push with your palm again.

6. Continue pushing and folding to knead for 5 to 10 minutes, until the dough is firm.

7. When the dough is smooth and elastic, shape it into a ball and place it in a clean, large bowl. Cover with foil or plastic wrap and set aside for 30 minutes. Make sure that the dough doesn't dry out.

8. Clear and clean a large, flat area. Separate the dough into 4 roughly equal sections, working with one section at a time.

9. On the prepared and liberally floured flat surface, roll the dough out into a rectangle. Keep it as thin as possible so that you can gently pick it up without it breaking, but at the same time, it is so thin that you're nearly able to see your fingers through the dough.

10. When formed, cut for the desired pasta size. Fettuccine should be cut about ¼-inch, while linguine is narrower and should be cut at ⅛-inch.

Fresh Veggie Noodles (continued)

11. As you cut them, pick up portions and shake them out to separate, ensuring that the pasta is fully cut. Toss with a small bit of flour to prevent sticking. Twirl loosely into mounds to rest as you continue through the entire quantity of dough.

to cook

1. Heat water and 2 teaspoons salt in a large saucepan or small stockpot and bring to a full boil.

2. Drop the desired portions of fresh pasta into the boiling water.

3. Cook the pasta for 2 to 5 minutes, depending on the thickness you cut. Taste to confirm doneness. The texture should be soft but not mushy.

4. When finished, use tongs to remove the pasta from the water.

to store

1. Pasta is best used immediately, but can be refrigerated for three to five days.

2. To freeze in portions, place the twirled mounds on a parchment paper-lined baking sheet and freeze for between 60 and 90 minutes. Remove from the freezer and transfer to a freezer bag or vacuum-sealed bag to store for up to 6 months. The first step of freezing prevents the strips from sticking together.

TIP: Rather use a food processor? Add the flour and salt to the bowl of a food processor and mix for 15 seconds to combine. Keep the food processor running and slowly add one egg at a time, allowing time for the liquid to fully combine before adding the second egg. Slowly add vegetable juice and olive oil in the same way. It will start to form large clumps, but will have loose flour bits. Transfer to the flat surface and continue the recipe instructions from the point of kneading.

Homemade Chicken Pot Pie

ingredients

2 individual pie crusts (homemade or frozen)

⅓ cup butter

½ cup minced celery

½ cup minced leeks or onion

4 chicken breasts, cut into quarters

1 ¾ cups chicken broth

⅓ cup all-purpose flour

1 can of cream of chicken soup (may substitute any "cream of")

½ cup whole milk

¼ teaspoon celery seed

3 cups riced carrots

½ cup puréed peas

Salt and pepper to taste

directions

1. Preheat oven to 425°F.

2. Place one pie crust (shell) into a 9-inch pie pan and bake until lightly browned.

3. Remove from oven and set aside. Reduce oven temperature to 300°F.

4. Warm the butter in a large saucepan over medium heat until it melts. Add the leeks or onions and celery and sauté until tender.

5. Add chicken breasts and chicken broth. Bring to a boil.

6. Reduce heat to a simmer and cook for 8 to 10 minutes.

7. In a medium bowl, mix flour, cream of chicken soup, and milk, whisking until there are no lumps.

8. Slowly pour this mixture over the chicken.

9. Add celery seed, salt, pepper, carrots, and peas and stir to combine.

10. Cook for 5 to 7 minutes, until thickened. Remove from heat.

11. Spoon into the baked shell until full. Lay the second crust over the top and crimp it into the baked shell.

12. Make several cuts in the crust to vent.

13. Bake for about 30 minutes until golden brown.

14. Remove from the oven and allow to rest for 10 to 15 minutes before serving.

Pumpkin Beef Stew

directions

1. Cut beef into 1-inch chunks.

2. Pat the beef dry to remove any excess moisture.

3. Mix the flour, nutmeg, salt, and pepper in a shallow pan or clean plastic storage bag.

4. Add the beef and toss until it is completely covered on all sides with the flavored flour. Press the beef lightly into the flour to make sure it adheres.

5. Heat the butter and olive oil at medium-high heat in a large stock pot. Add the beef in small batches and cook, browning it on all sides. Set aside the cooked beef.

6. Add minced garlic and leeks to the pot and sauté for 1 to 2 minutes.

7. Add beef stock, pumpkin purée, and Worcestershire sauce and stir.

8. Bring to a boil, then reduce the heat and simmer for 3 hours, stirring occasionally.

9. Add the potatoes, rutabaga, carrots, and peas.

10. Increase the heat to medium and cook for 30 to 35 minutes.

11. Serve immediately in individual bowls with bread or rolls.

ingredients

3 lbs of beef (stew meat or chuck roast)

½ cup all-purpose flour

1 teaspoon ground nutmeg

1 tablespoon salt

1 teaspoon ground black pepper

2 tablespoons butter

1 tablespoon olive oil

1 garlic clove, minced

1 cup diced leeks

4 cups beef stock or broth

2 cups pumpkin purée

1 tablespoon Worcestershire sauce

2 lbs of potatoes, peeled and diced

1 lb of rutabaga, peeled and diced

4 cups diced carrots

½ cup puréed green peas

Veggie Peanut Chicken and Zucchini Noodles

ingredients

2 cups water

2 cups chicken or vegetable stock

2 large chicken breasts, quartered

2 whole carrots, peeled and chopped into 2- to 3-inch pieces

1 large red bell pepper, seeds removed and quartered.

1 jalapeño, halved and seeds removed (optional)

1 tablespoon olive oil

2 teaspoons minced garlic

½ cup minced leeks

3 large zucchini, spiralized into noodles

ingredients: sauce

⅓ cup honey

⅓ cup soy sauce

2 tablespoons sesame oil

2 tablespoons rice vinegar

1 teaspoon ginger

½ cup creamy peanut butter

1 tablespoon sesame seeds

1 tablespoon dried cilantro

½ cup chopped peanuts

½ cup riced Brussels sprouts

1 teaspoon hot sauce

directions

1. In a large saucepan over medium heat, add water, vegetable stock, and chicken.

2. Add, carrots, bell peppers, and jalapeño.

3. Boil for 8 to 10 minutes. Remove from heat.

4. Using a strainer placed over a large pot, drain off the liquid.

5. Place the chicken on a plate to cool, then shred. Set aside.

6. Add all of the vegetables to a food processor along with a ½ cup of the liquid. Discard the remaining liquid. Pulse the vegetables on high until puréed. Set aside.

7. Warm olive oil in a large skillet. Add garlic and leeks and sauté until tender. Add the **zucchini noodles** and shredded chicken to the skillet.

8. Cook and stir for about 3 minutes until the chicken is warm and the zucchini is slightly soft, but not mushy. Remove from heat.

9. In a medium saucepan over low heat, mix the honey, soy sauce, sesame oil, rice vinegar, ginger, and peanut butter. Whisk constantly until the peanut butter has melted and the mixture is smooth.

10. Add the vegetable purée, sesame seeds, cilantro, peanuts, Brussels sprouts, and hot sauce. Heat for 2 to 3 minutes.

11. Pour the sauce over the chicken and zucchini noodles.

12. Toss until combined.

13. Serve immediately.

TIP: If you test this recipe and don't like the zucchini noodles, follow the same instructions, substituting cooked linguini for the zucchini noodles. The sauce is still chock-full of other hidden veggies!

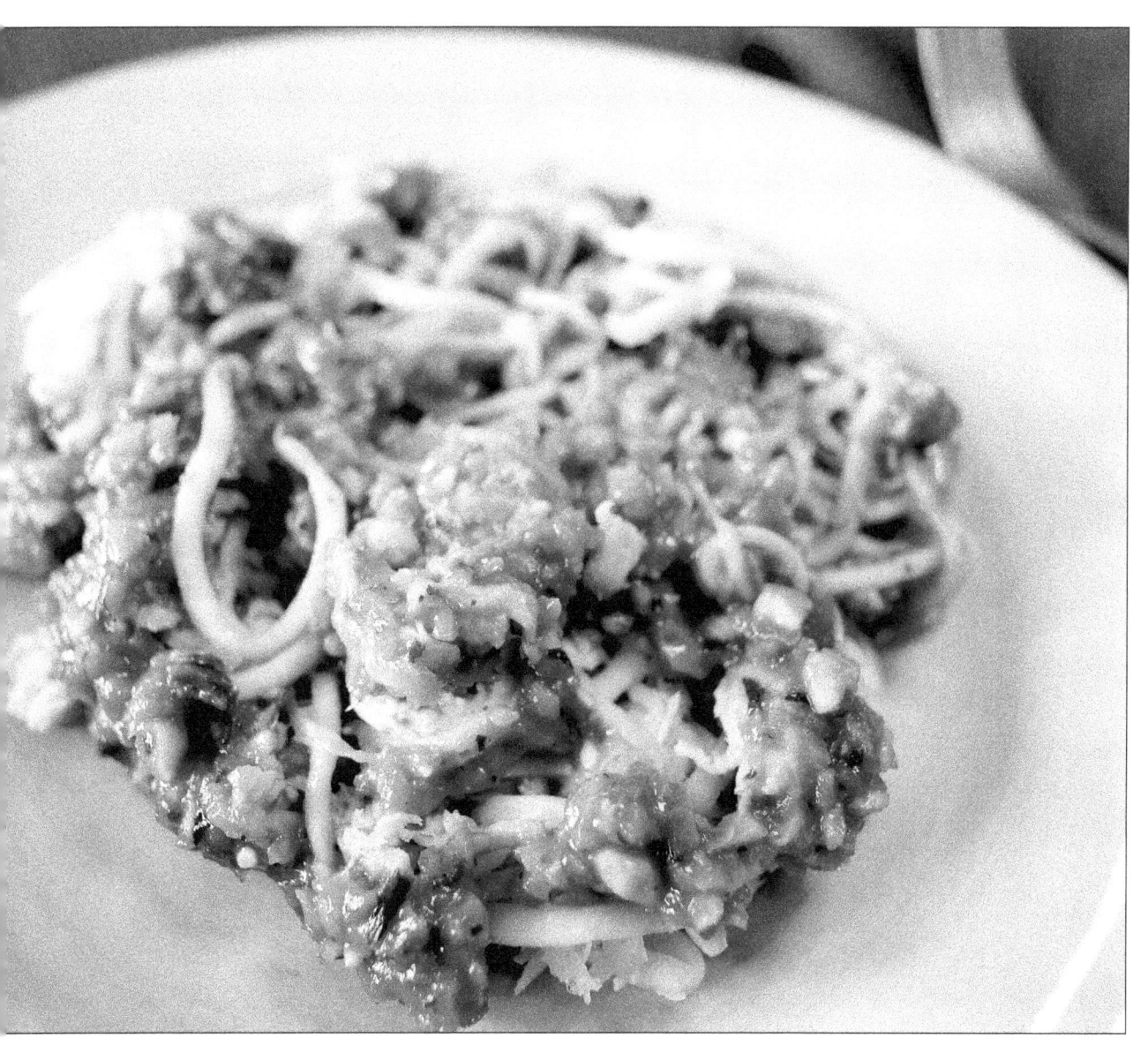

Shepherd's Pie

ingredients

Premade pie crust (or use homemade)

1 large rutabaga, peeled and cubed

½ teaspoon salt (divided)

½ teaspoon pepper (divided)

2 teaspoons granulated garlic (divided)

2 tablespoons margarine

¼ cup milk

1 lb of ground beef

1 tablespoon flour

1 cup minced leeks or onion

2 tablespoons Worcestershire sauce

½ teaspoon red pepper

½ teaspoon paprika

1 package frozen peas and carrot mix

One 15-ounce can of cream-style corn

1 minced red bell pepper

directions

1. Preheat oven to 350°F.

2. Place the crust in a 9-inch pie pan.

3. Place the chopped rutabaga in a large pot and cover with cold, salted water. Bring to a boil and cook for 20 to 25 minutes or until tender.

4. Drain and press the rutabaga with a potato masher until it reaches the desired consistency. Add 1 teaspoon garlic powder, ¼ teaspoon salt, ¼ teaspoon pepper, margarine, and milk, mixing until smooth. Set aside.

5. Cook the ground beef in a large skillet over medium heat until browned. Drain excess fat.

6. Return the skillet to heat and stir in the flour.

7. Add leeks or onion, Worcestershire sauce, red pepper, paprika, and the remaining salt, pepper, and garlic.

8. Simmer for 5 minutes on low heat. Remove from heat and cool.

9. Place the frozen peas and carrot mix in a food processor and pulse to rice-sized pieces.

10. In a large bowl, combine the peas and carrots, cream-style corn, and minced bell pepper. Add the cooled meat mixture to it and stir to combine.

11. Spoon into the bottom of the pie shell (crust).

12. Spread the mashed rutabaga so that it covers the top of the meat pie.

13. Bake for 30 minutes, or until the pie crust and top are a golden brown.

14. Serve immediately.

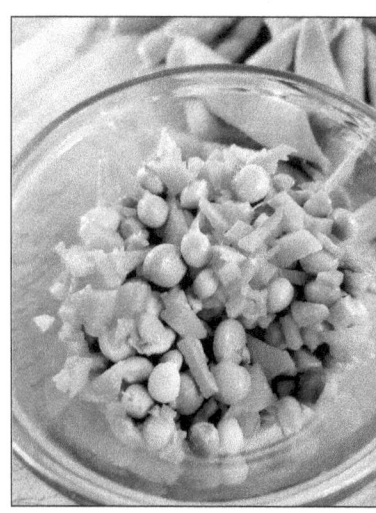

Fresh peas and carrot mix.

Pepperoni Spinach Roll-Up

directions

1. In a large bowl, mix sauce, **spinach purée,** garlic powder, and onion powder until smooth.

2. Roll out the bread dough as a 12-inch square.

3. Spread about ½ the sauce over the dough in a thin layer. Reserve the excess sauce.

4. Lay pepperoni over the dough, overlapping the edges to cover completely.

5. Top with shredded cheese.

6. Roll up the dough square and place on a baking sheet.

7. Cover with a clean towel and set aside to proof for about 30 to 45 minutes.

8. Preheat oven to 375°F.

9. In a small microwave-safe bowl, melt 1 tablespoon of the butter. Brush lightly over the dough before baking.

10. Bake for 18 to 20 minutes or until golden brown.

11. In the same bowl, melt the remaining 2 tablespoons of butter, then add the Italian seasoning, garlic powder, and Parmesan cheese to it, whisking to blend. Brush over the top of the bread immediately upon removing the roll-up from the oven.

12. Allow it to rest for 5 minutes before slicing.

13. Serve with the sauce reserved for dipping.

ingredients

3 cups spaghetti or pizza sauce

½ cup **spinach purée**

1 teaspoon garlic powder

½ teaspoon onion powder

1 loaf of bread dough, defrosted if frozen

One 6-ounce packet of pepperoni

1½ cups shredded mozzarella cheese

3 tablespoons melted butter

1 teaspoon Italian seasoning

½ teaspoon garlic powder

1 tablespoon Parmesan cheese

Chicken Tetrazzini with Asparagus

ingredients

2 cups water

1 cup dry white wine

1½ teaspoons pepper, divided

1 teaspoon garlic powder

2 boneless, skinless chicken breasts, quartered

One 16-ounce packet of linguine or fettuccine

1 can cream of chicken with herbs soup

1 can cream of asparagus soup

2 cups sour cream

½ cup unsalted butter, softened

1 cup chicken broth

1 cup riced carrots

1 cup minced asparagus

1 teaspoon parsley flakes

2 cups shredded mozzarella cheese

2 tablespoons grated Parmesan cheese

directions

1. Place the chicken breasts in a medium stock pot with water, white wine, pepper, and garlic powder.

2. Bring the liquid to a boil, then reduce the heat to low. Cover and simmer for about 15 minutes, or until fully cooked.

3. Remove the chicken. Set aside to cool.

4. Preheat the oven to 350°F.

5. Spray a 9 x13 baking dish with non-stick spray and set aside.

6. Cook pasta according to the box instructions. Drain and set aside.

7. In a large bowl, mix the two cans of soup, sour cream, butter, pepper, and chicken broth.

8. Stir in riced carrots and asparagus.

9. Shred the cooled chicken and add to the mixture. Add cooked noodles and blend until fully coated.

10. Spoon into the prepared baking dish.

11. Evenly spread mozzarella cheese on top, then sprinkle Parmesan.

12. Bake for 35 to 45 minutes, until the cheeses are melted and lightly browned.

13. Serve immediately.

TIP Save time: Start with rotisserie chicken and have the meal prep done in minutes!

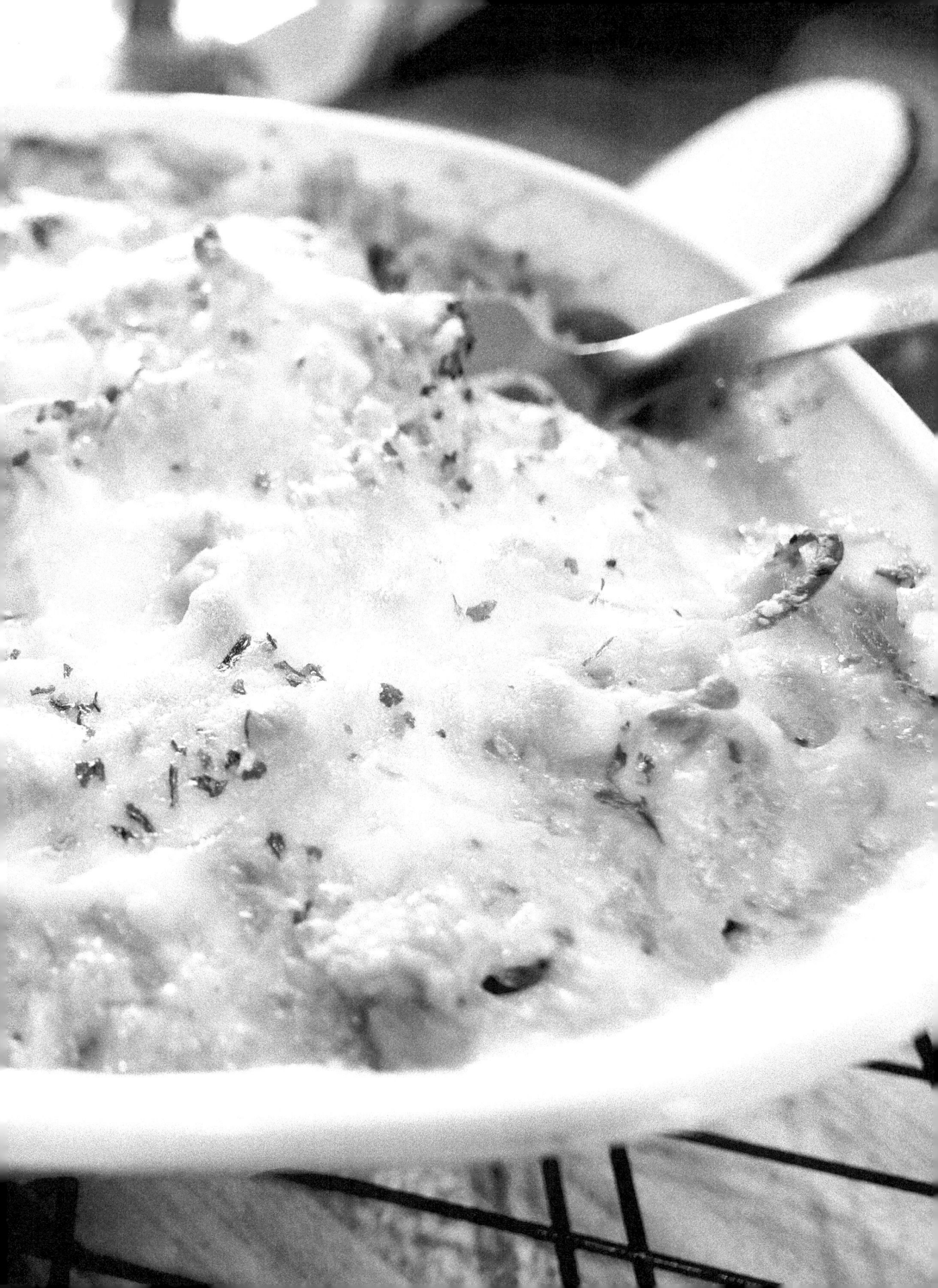

Skillet Ziti with Sausage & Kale

ingredients

1 lb of lean ground beef or Italian sausage

1 teaspoon olive oil

1 cup minced leeks or onion

4 garlic cloves, minced

2½ cups roasted cherry tomatoes

½ cup kale purée

½ teaspoon red pepper flakes

1 teaspoon tomato paste

One 16-ounce box of dry ziti pasta

3 cups water

½ cup grated Parmesan cheese

1 tablespoon dried basil (or 4 tablespoons fresh basil)

½ teaspoon salt

¼ teaspoon pepper

1 cup mozzarella cheese, shredded

directions

1. In a deep, oven-safe skillet, brown the ground beef or Italian sausage until no pink remains.

2. Remove and set aside on a paper towel-lined plate to drain excess grease.

3. Add 1 teaspoon olive oil to the skillet. Sauté leeks or onion and garlic on medium for 2 to 3 minutes or until tender.

4. Increase heat to medium-high. Add cherry tomato, kale purée, red pepper flakes, and tomato paste. Stir to combine.

5. Add water and dry pasta.

6. Bring to a boil, then reduce heat to low. Cover and simmer, stirring occasionally, for 15 to 18 minutes or until the pasta is tender.

7. Add additional hot water if necessary.

8. Add the ground beef/Italian sausage and Parmesan. Stir in basil, salt, and pepper. Cook on low for 2 to 3 minutes.

9. Remove from heat.

10. Spread mozzarella evenly on top.

11. Set the oven to broil.

12. Place the skillet in the oven and broil for about 5 minutes, until the cheese is browned and bubbling.

13. Serve immediately.

Stuffed Pasta Shells

directions

1. In a large skillet, cook the sausage until browned. Drain fat.

2. Add the **bell pepper** and garlic to the sausage and cook for 2 to 3 minutes, until the bell pepper is softened.

3. Add spaghetti sauce, oregano, and basil, stirring to combine. Remove from heat and set aside.

4. In a large saucepan, boil water and prepare pasta shells according to package instructions. Drain and cool.

5. Preheat oven to 350°F.

6. In a 9x12 baking dish, pour a small amount of spaghetti sauce, just enough to cover the surface.

7. In a large bowl, combine the Ricotta cheese, **puréed kale,** nutmeg, and ½ cup of mozzarella cheese. Stir to combine.

8. Scoop the cheese and kale mixture using a tablespoon to fill each shell.

9. Place in the prepared baking dish. Repeat until the entire cheese mixture is used and the shells are filled.

10. Pour the remaining sauce on top of the stuffed shells and cover with the remaining mozzarella cheese.

11. Bake for 45 minutes. Check after 30 minutes. If the cheese is getting too browned, cover with foil and continue cooking.

12. Serve warm.

ingredients

1 lb of mild or spicy Italian sausage

1 cup **minced bell pepper**

2 garlic cloves, minced

1 jar spaghetti sauce

½ teaspoon oregano

½ teaspoon basil

Cooking Spray

1 box of pasta shells, cooked

15 ounce part skim Ricotta cheese

2 cups **puréed kale**

1 teaspoon nutmeg

1 cup shredded mozzarella cheese

Sloppy Joes

ingredients

1 tablespoon olive oil

½ cup minced leeks or onion

1 garlic clove, minced

¼ cup minced celery

½ cup riced carrot

1 lb of ground beef

One 15-ounce can tomato sauce or ½ cup ketchup

¼ cup brown sugar

1½ teaspoons chili powder

½ teaspoon salt

½ teaspoon pepper

1 teaspoon apple cider vinegar

1 teaspoon yellow mustard

directions

1. Warm olive oil in a large skillet over medium heat. Add the leeks or onion, garlic, celery, and carrots and sauté for 2 to 3 minutes or until softened.

2. Add the ground beef and cook until the meat has browned all the way through. Drain the excess fat.

3. Add the tomato sauce (or ketchup), brown sugar, chili powder, salt, pepper, vinegar, and mustard.

4. Simmer over low heat for about 10 to 15 minutes, until the sauce thickens.

5. Serve on hamburger buns, kaiser rolls, or Spinach Buns (p. 80).

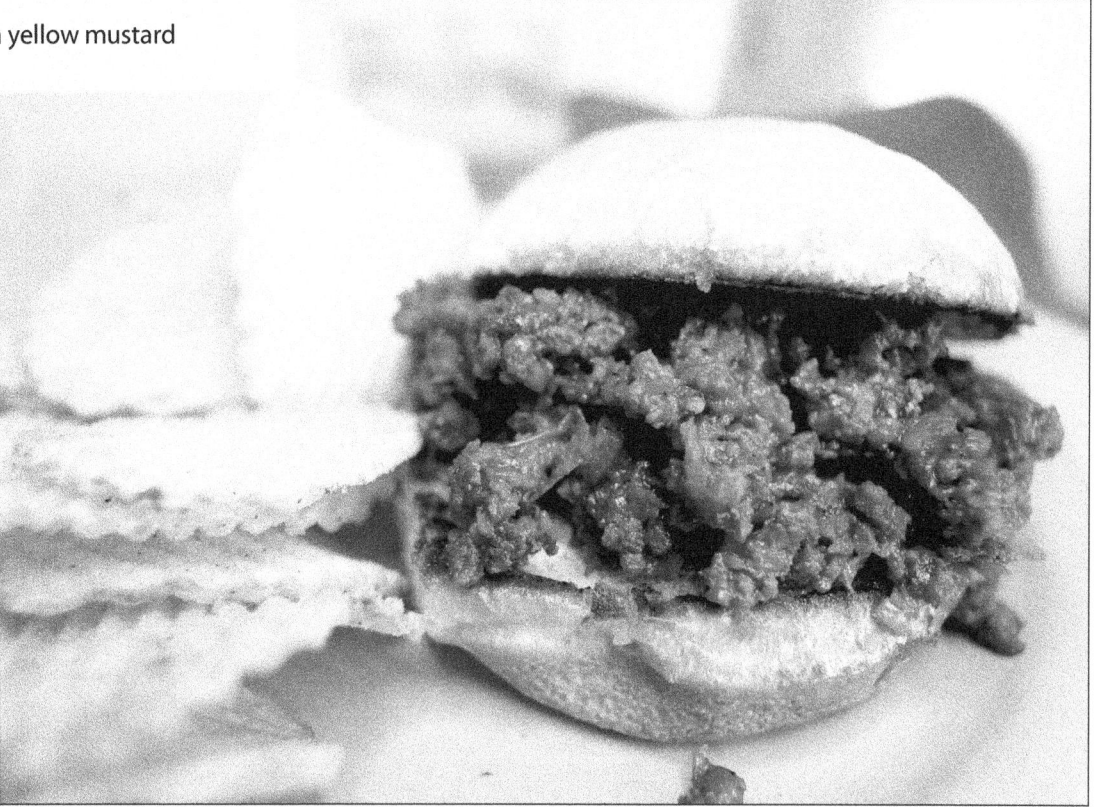

Crock Pot Pasta Bolognese-style Sauce

directions

1. Warm 1 tablespoon olive oil in a large skillet over high heat. Add garlic and leeks or onion, cooking for 5 to 7 minutes or until the vegetables are translucent.

2. Add beef or sausage and continue cooking until the meat is browned all the way through. Transfer cooked meat to a slow cooker on low.

3. Return the skillet to the stove over medium heat and add 1 tablespoon olive oil, red wine, and crushed beef bouillon, whisking to blend.

4. Bring to a simmer while continuing to whisk, keeping the mixture smooth.

5. Add the **puréed beets,** tomato paste, Worcestershire sauce, oregano, thyme leaves, bay leaves, red pepper flakes, salt, and pepper. Simmer the mixture for 5 minutes, whisking to keep it smooth and prevent burning.

6. Transfer the sauce from the skillet to a slow cooker, add tomatoes and celery.

7. Cook on low for 6 hours.

8. Serve over pasta.

TIP: For a stronger flavor kick, substitute the crushed tomato with an equal amount of Rotel.

ingredients

- 2 tablespoons olive oil (divided)
- 4 garlic cloves, crushed
- 2 cups minced leeks or onions
- ½ cup minced celery
- 2 lbs of ground beef or Italian sausage
- 1 cup red wine or beef broth
- 3 beef bouillon cubes, crushed
- ¼ cup **puréed beets**
- 4 tablespoons tomato paste
- 2 teaspoons Worcestershire Sauce
- 3 teaspoons dried oregano
- 2 teaspoons dried thyme leaves
- 3 dried bay leaves
- 2 teaspoons red pepper flakes
- 1 teaspoon salt
- ½ teaspoon pepper
- Two 28-ounce canned crushed tomatoes, or 20 whole fresh tomatoes with skins and seeds removed

Western Beef and Corn Casserole

ingredients: filling

1 lb of ground beef

¼ cup diced leeks or onion

½ teaspoon salt

½ teaspoon chili powder

1 cup Fiesta Corn (see p. 132)

1 cup Smooth Salsa (see p. 61) or 1 cup of your favorite salsa, enchilada sauce, or taco sauce

½ cup shredded cheddar cheese

ingredients: crust

½ cup all-purpose flour

½ cup yellow cornmeal

½ cup riced cauliflower

2 tablespoons sugar

1 teaspoon salt

1 teaspoon baking powder

¼ cup cold butter

½ cup milk

1 egg, lightly beaten

1 cup shredded cheddar cheese, divided

Photo opposite page.

directions

1. Preheat oven to 400°F.

2. Spray a 9-inch square baking dish with non-stick cooking oil. Set aside.

3. In a large skillet, cook beef with leeks or onion, salt, and chili powder over medium heat until the meat has browned all the way through. Drain the excess fat.

4. Stir in Fiesta Corn, salsa, and shredded cheese. Set aside.

5. In a large bowl, combine the flour, cornmeal, cauliflower, sugar, salt, and baking powder.

6. Using a pastry cutter, cut in the butter until the mixture resembles coarse crumbs.

7. Add milk and egg. Stir until combined.

8. Add ½ cup cheddar cheese.

9. Press the crust mixture into the prepared baking dish, covering the bottom and sides of the dish.

10. Spoon the meat mixture into the crust and top with the remaining cheese.

11. Bake for 20 to 25 minutes or until the cheese is lightly browned and bubbly.

12. Serve warm.

Sausage & Kohlrabi Fettuccini

directions

1. Cook the pasta according to the package directions.

2. In a large skillet, cook sausage over medium heat until fully cooked and lightly browned. Remove the sausage and set aside.

3. Return the skillet to the stove and reset the heat to medium. Add olive oil and heat for one minute. Add minced garlic and **minced kohlrabi** and sauté for 1 to 2 minutes.

4. Add cream, paprika, cayenne pepper, salt, pepper, and nutmeg. Bring to a boil, stirring occasionally.

5. Add Parmesan cheese and reduce heat.

6. Simmer for 3 to 4 minutes until the mixture begins to thicken.

7. Add the sausage to the skillet and simmer for 2 minutes more.

8. Serve over the fettuccini noodles.

ingredients

One 16-ounce package Fettuccini OR 8 cups homemade Fettuccini (see p. 118)

One 14-ounce package of smoked sausage cut into ¼-inch slices

2 tablespoons olive oil

1–2 garlic cloves, minced

1 cup **minced kohlrabi**

2 cups heavy cream

1 teaspoon dried oregano

1 teaspoon paprika

1 teaspoon cayenne pepper

½ teaspoon salt or to taste

½ teaspoon ground black pepper

½ teaspoon nutmeg

½ cup fresh grated Parmesan cheese

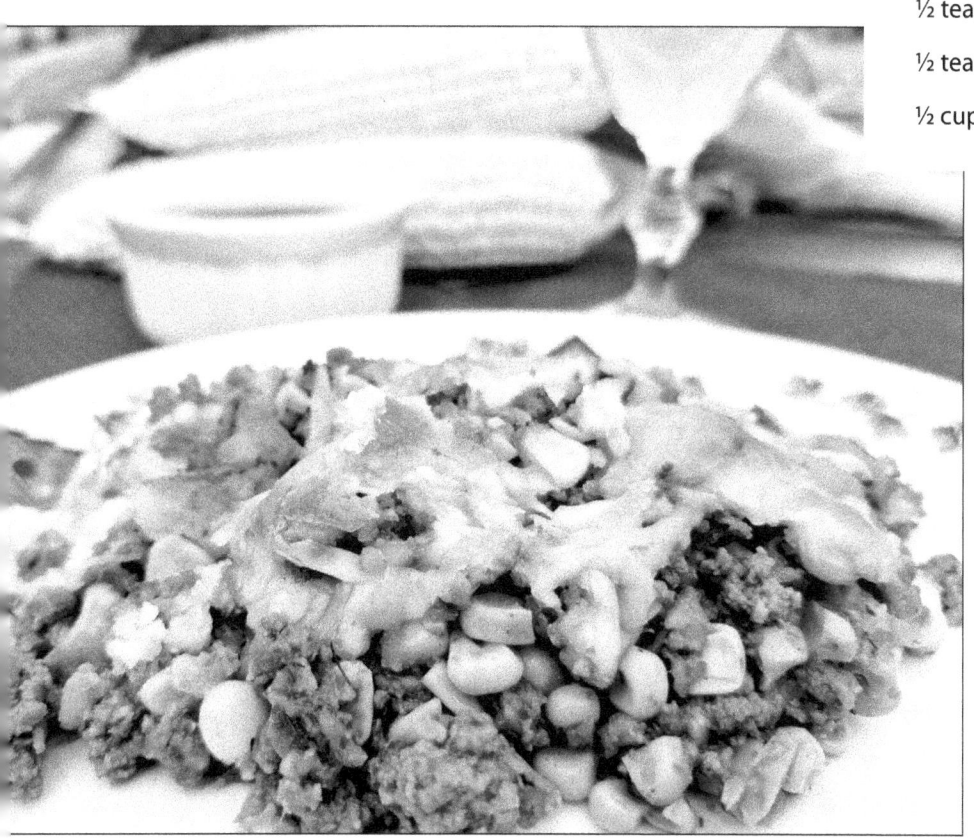

Western Beef and Corn Casserole recipe opposite page.

Main Dishes

Fresh vs Frozen

Fresh Vegetables

PROs

Nutrition If freshly-picked, they're packed with nutrient.

Flexible Buying vegetables fresh typically gives you more of the vegetable, like leaves or stems.

Additives Buying fresh allows you certainty that there are no hidden ingredients or additives, as long as you wash them fully.

CONs

Nutrient Fade Nutrients are lost if they're not stored properly.

Quick Spoilage They can spoil fast, so it's best to use them quickly.

Costly Choices Fresh produce can be pricier, especially when it's out of season.

Prep-Time Fresh produce requires extra time for cleaning, peeling, and prepping.

Availability Some vegetables are only readily available at certain times of the year.

Frozen Vegetables

PROs

Nutrient Preservation Frozen veggies are often picked at peak ripeness and flash-frozen to lock in the nutrition.

Last Longer They have a longer shelf life, helping reduce food waste.

Convenience Many frozen veggies come pre-washed and pre-cut, saving time in prep work.

Budget-Friendly Often, frozen vegetables are more affordable than fresh ones, especially in off-seasons.

Availability You can find a variety of frozen veggies year-round.

CONs

Texture The freezing process changes the texture of some vegetables, making them mushy or mealy. Asparagus is one that doesn't hold up well after being frozen.

Additives Sugar, salt, spices, as well as chemicals or preservatives may be added, so always check the labels.

Limited Choices Grocery stores may have a limited selection of frozen vegetables.

Thaw/Refreeze During the shipping and storage process, frozen food may thaw and refreeze, with impacts that range from undesirable consistency to contamination.

photo opposite page: © Scott Erb & Donna Dufault – www.erbphoto.com

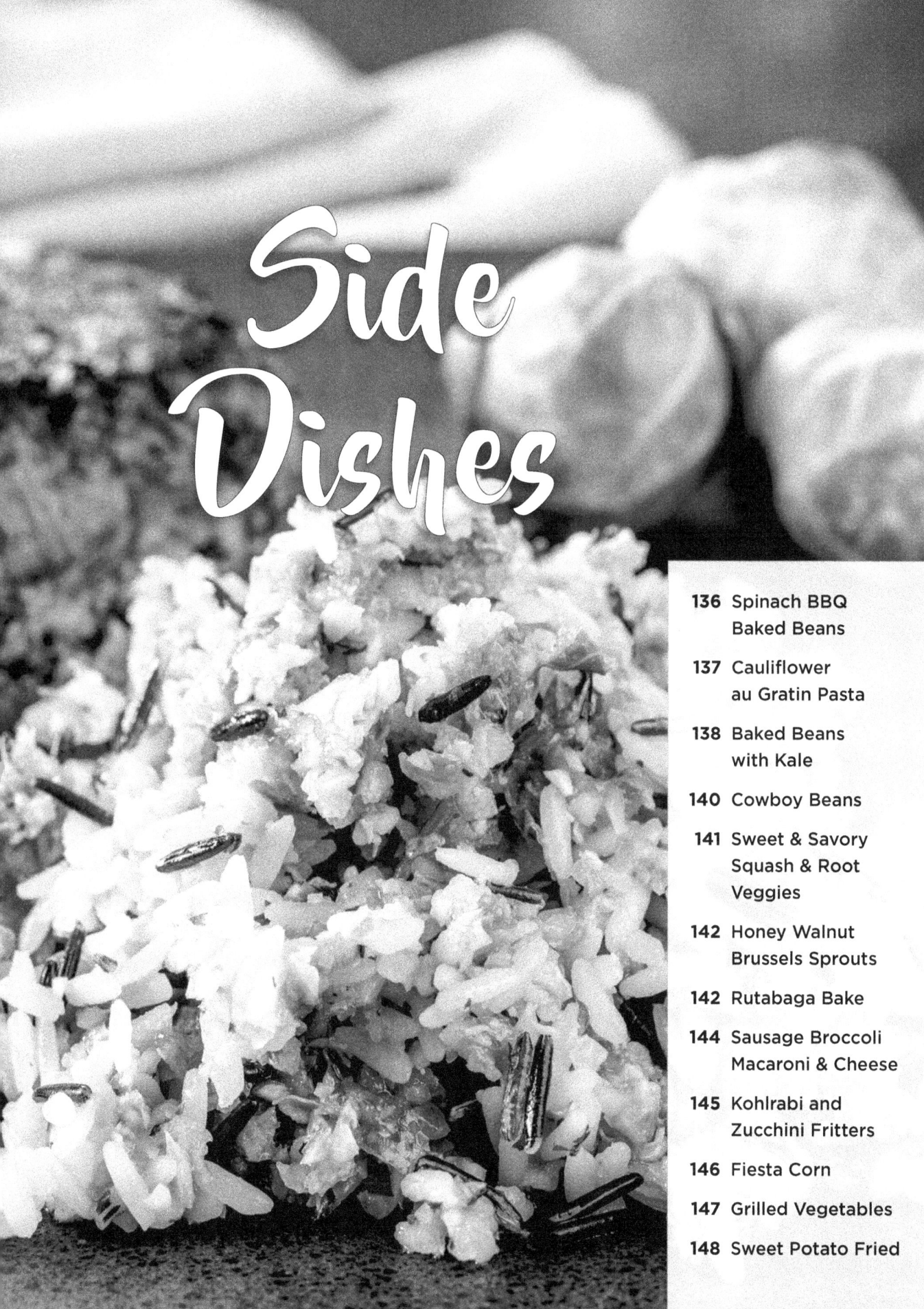

Side Dishes

- **136** Spinach BBQ Baked Beans
- **137** Cauliflower au Gratin Pasta
- **138** Baked Beans with Kale
- **140** Cowboy Beans
- **141** Sweet & Savory Squash & Root Veggies
- **142** Honey Walnut Brussels Sprouts
- **142** Rutabaga Bake
- **144** Sausage Broccoli Macaroni & Cheese
- **145** Kohlrabi and Zucchini Fritters
- **146** Fiesta Corn
- **147** Grilled Vegetables
- **148** Sweet Potato Fried

Spinach BBQ Baked Beans

ingredients

4 slices bacon

1 tablespoon olive oil

1 garlic clove, minced

1 fresh jalapeño, diced (optional)

1 cup **puréed spinach**

½ cup barbecue sauce

½ cup water

2 tablespoons tomato paste

¼ cup brown sugar

1 tablespoon white vinegar

⅛ teaspoon salt

¼ teaspoon pepper

¼ teaspoon chili powder

Two 15-ounce cans of great northern beans (drained and rinsed)

directions

1. Preheat oven to 350°F.

2. In a deep skillet or large saucepan, cook bacon until crispy. Cool and crumble, then set aside.

3. Drain bacon grease and add olive oil to the skillet.

4. Add garlic and jalapeño and cook for 3 to 4 minutes. Remove from heat.

5. In a large bowl, whisk together **puréed spinach,** barbeque sauce, water, tomato paste, brown sugar, vinegar, salt, pepper, and chili powder.

6. Add the garlic and jalapeno.

7. Add the beans and crumbled bacon. Mix to blend.

8. Spoon into a 9-inch square baking dish.

9. Bake for 50 to 60 minutes.

10. Serve warm.

Cauliflower au Gratin Pasta

directions

1. Preheat the oven to 350°F.
2. Using a medium saucepan, prepare pasta according to the package directions.
3. Drain and place the pasta in a baking dish. Mix in riced cauliflower and minced asparagus.
4. Using the same saucepan, melt butter and add the flour, whisking to prevent burning. Slowly whisk in the milk until a thin sauce forms.
5. Add the Dijon mustard, salt, pepper, and half the cheese. Stir until the cheese melts and the sauce is smooth.
6. Pour the sauce over the pasta mix.
7. Spread the remaining cheese on top and bake for 10 to 15 minutes until the cheese melts and is lightly browned.
8. Serve warm.

TIP: For a more flavorful dish, don't be afraid to use stronger cheese or add your favorite spices! Try chili powder for spice, nutmeg or ginger for savory, or diced jalapeños for heat.

ingredients

16 ounce dry uncooked pasta (ziti, rotini, or bowtie)

1 cup riced cauliflower

1 cup minced asparagus

4 tablespoons butter

½ cup flour

4 cups milk

1 tablespoon Dijon mustard

½ teaspoon salt

½ teaspoon pepper

1½ cups shredded sharp cheddar cheese

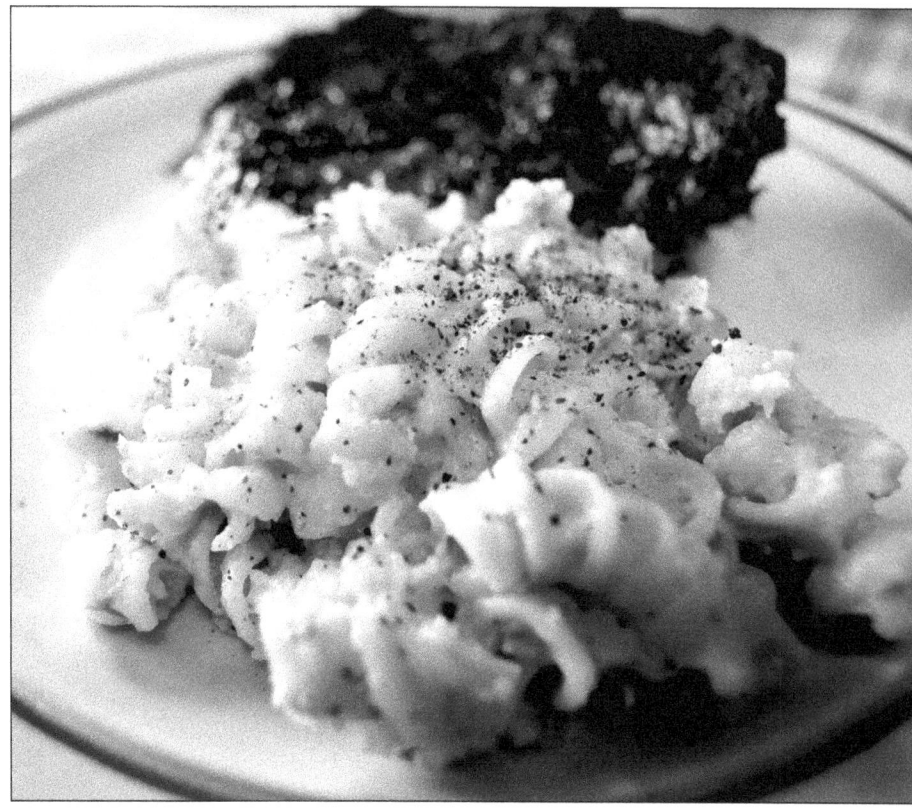

Baked Beans with Kale

ingredients

2⅓ cups dry great northern beans (1# bag)

1 cup ketchup

½ cup barbecue sauce

⅓ cup brown sugar

2 tablespoons yellow mustard

¼ cup white vinegar

3 tablespoons chili powder

1 cup **puréed kale**

½ cup minced leeks or onion

directions

1. Prepare beans according to the package directions. For a quick version of this, use canned beans.

2. Preheat oven to 350°F.

3. In a large bowl, combine ketchup, barbecue sauce, brown sugar, mustard, vinegar, chili powder, puréed kale, and leeks or onions. Add the beans and stir to combine.

4. Spoon into a casserole dish.

5. Bake uncovered for 1 hour.

6. Serve warm.

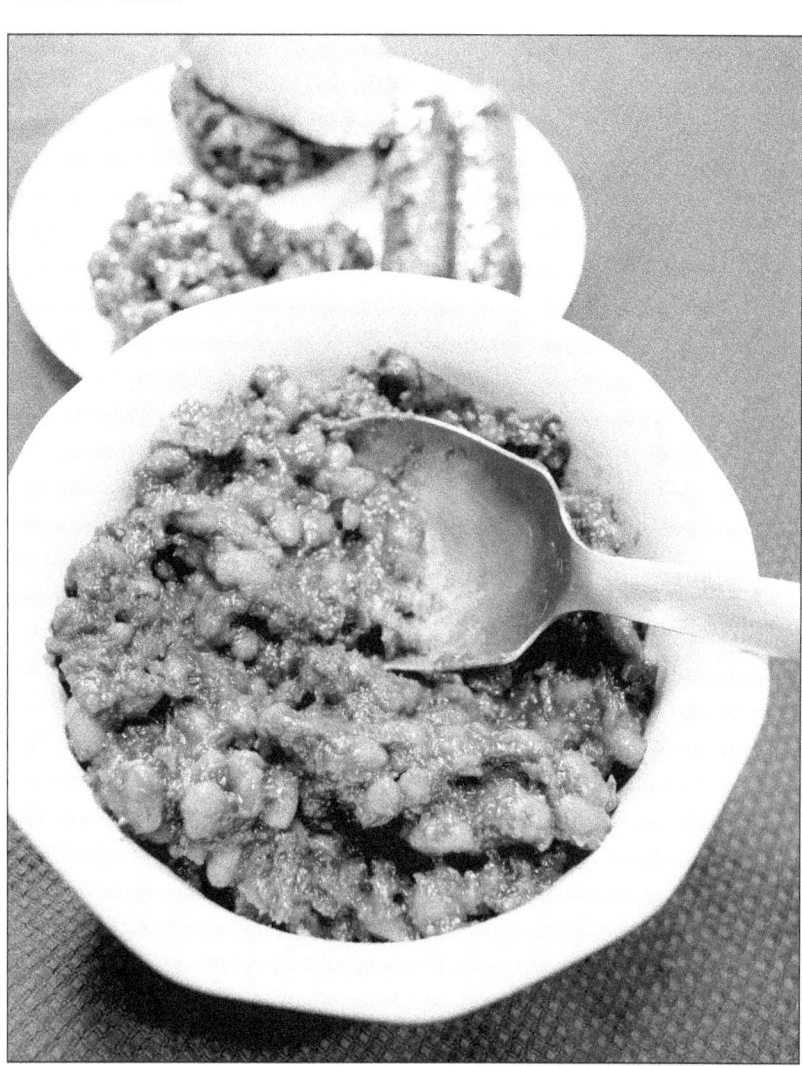

Fast Veggie-Infused Side Dishes

In a hurry and need fast veggie-infused main or side dishes? Start with canned or frozen convenience foods and add riced, minced, or pureed veggies from the Core, plus spices and flavor enhancers. Below are suggestions—use some but not all. Use flavors you like and disguise those you don't. Start small and see what you like. Have fun with experimentation!

Start with	Add Veggie	Add spice and Flavor option(s)
Long Grain Rice	Minced carrots or minced asparagus	Garlic, onion, parsley, thyme, vegetable broth
Spanish/Mexican Rice	Minced leeks/onion, minced carrots	Chili powder, garlic, cilantro
Canned or Frozen Corn	FOR SWEET: pureed sweet potato, pureed butternut squash	Cinnamon, ginger, nutmeg, butter, honey
Canned or Frozen Corn	FOR SAVORY: minced leeks or onion, minced carrot	Garlic, paprika, salt, pepper, cheese
Canned Pork & Beans	Pureed spinach, pureed kale, minced carrot, minced leeks or onion	Chili powder, cayenne, salt, pepper, apple cider vinegar
Macaroni & Cheese	Riced cauliflower or minced broccoli	Chili powder or ground mustard
Au Gratin Potatoes	Minced leeks/onions, minced carrots, minced broccoli	Thyme, nutmeg, garlic, pepper, paprika, cayenne
Scalloped Potatoes	Minced carrots, minced broccoli	Garlic, thyme, nutmeg, pepper, bacon bits
Mashed Potatoes	Riced cauliflower, minced leeks or onion, pureed butternut or acorn squash	Garlic, salt, pepper, chives, parsley, sage, paprika
Hashbrowns	Minced leeks/onions, minced carrots, minced bell pepper	Garlic, salt, pepper, paprika, chives, parsley
Corn Bread Mix	FOR SWEET: riced cauliflower, pureed butternut or acorn squash	Cinnamon, nutmeg, ginger, vanilla
Corn Bread Mix	FOR SAVORY: Minced bell pepper, minced jalapeno	Cumin, cayenne, garlic, chili powder
Chili	Minced leeks/onions, minced bell pepper, minced carrots, pureed beets, pureed spinach	Chili powder, cumin, cayenne, garlic, oregano, salt, pepper, white vinegar
Spaghetti Sauce	Minced leeks/onions, minced carrots, pureed beets, pureed spinach, minced celery	Oregano, Italian blend spice, salt, pepper, red wine vinegar
Gravy	Pureed beets, pureed spinach, pureed kale, minced leeks or minced onion	Pepper, garlic, beef stock
Canned Soup	Cauliflower water, Zucchini water	Salt, pepper, paprika
Canned Tuna	Minced leeks/onions, minced carrots, minced celery, minced bell pepper	Chili powder, garlic, salt, pepper, ginger, soy
Couscous	Minced leeks or onion, minced carrot, minced kohlrabi, pureed squash, minced broccoli	Curry, turmeric, cinnamon, cumin
Quinoa	Shredded zucchini, pureed sweet potato, minced tomato, pureed kale, pureed spinach	Curry, cilantro, chili powder, paprika, vinaigrette

Cowboy Beans

ingredients

1 lb of ground beef

½ cup diced leeks or onion

2 garlic cloves, minced

½ lb of bacon, cooked crisp and crumbled

Two 15-ounce cans of kidney beans, drained

One 15-ounce can of pork and beans, drained

One 15-ounce can of pinto beans, drained

1 diced jalapeño (seeds removed)

¾ cup riced Brussels sprouts

¾ cup **spinach purée**

1 cup barbecue sauce

½ cup ketchup

¼ cup brown sugar

3 tablespoons yellow mustard

2 tablespoons apple cider vinegar

2 tablespoons chili powder

1 teaspoon salt

1 teaspoon pepper

directions

1. Preheat oven to 350° F.

2. In a large skillet over medium heat, brown the ground beef until no longer pink. Drain any fat.

3. Add garlic and leeks or onion. Cook for 2 to 3 minutes more.

4. Combine the cooked ground beef, crumbled bacon, beans, jalapeño, and Brussels sprouts in a large bowl.

5. In a medium bowl, blend **spinach purée,** barbecue sauce, ketchup, brown sugar, mustard, vinegar, chili powder, salt, and pepper. Whisk until smooth.

6. Add the sauce to the ground beef and beans. Stir to mix completely.

7. Spoon into a 2 ½ quart baking dish.

8. Bake in the oven for 60 to 75 minutes.

9. Serve warm.

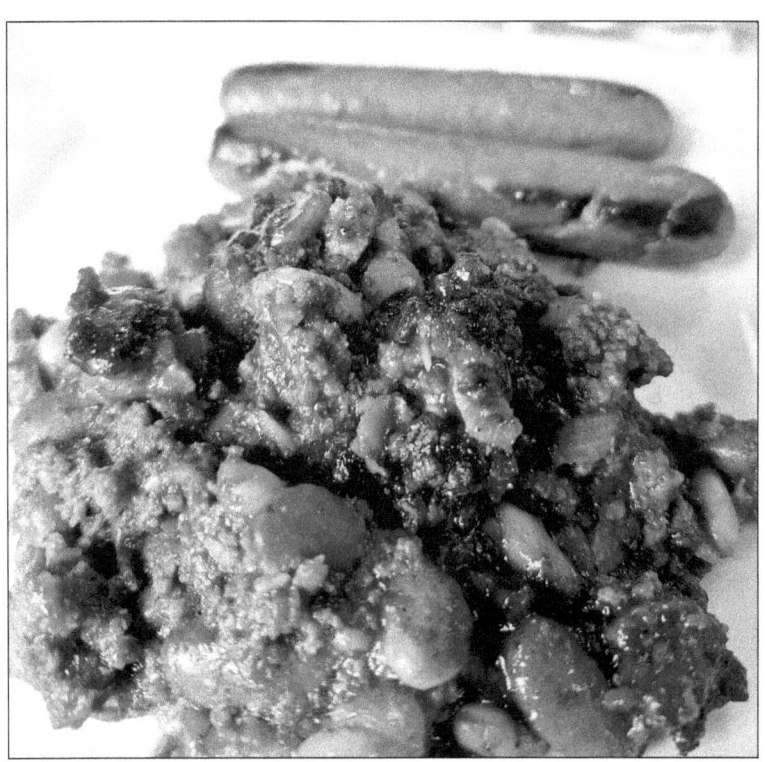

Sweet & Savory Squash & Root Veggies

directions

1. Preheat the oven to 425° F.
2. Line a large baking sheet with foil.
3. Add the diced vegetables to a large bowl. Set aside.
4. In a medium bowl, mix the olive oil, honey, brown sugar, thyme, rosemary, cinnamon, cayenne pepper, salt, and black pepper.
5. Pour the sauce over the vegetables and stir to coat thoroughly.
6. Spread the vegetables evenly onto the prepared baking sheet in a single layer.
7. Bake for 45 minutes, or until the veggies are tender and have slightly crispy edges. Remove from the oven.
8. Serve immediately.

ingredients

2 sweet potatoes, peeled and chopped into 1-inch cubes

1 butternut squash, peeled and chopped into 1-inch cubes

1 rutabaga, peeled and chopped into 1-inch cubes

3 cups **roasted beets**, chopped into 1-inch cubes

2 tablespoons olive oil

2 teaspoons honey

1 tablespoon brown sugar

1 tablespoon dried thyme

1 teaspoon rosemary

1 teaspoon paprika

½ teaspoon ground cinnamon

½ teaspoon salt

¼ teaspoon black pepper

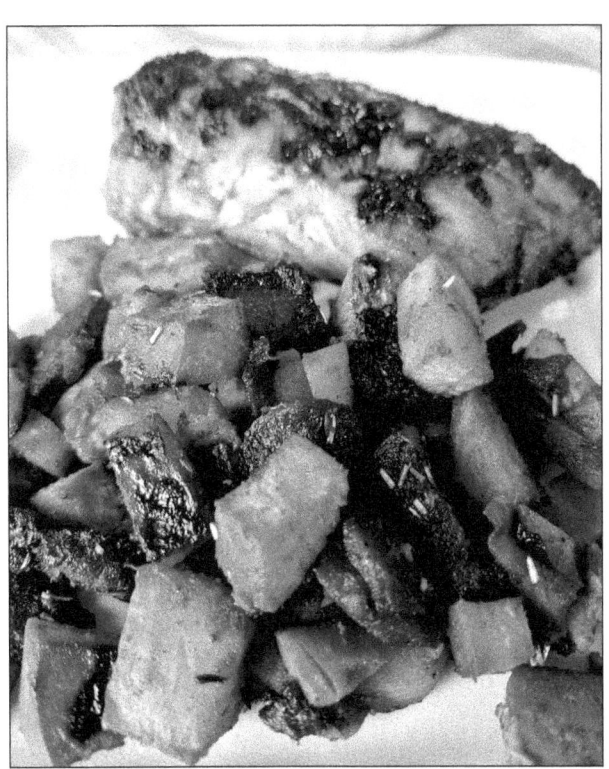

Side Dishes

Honey Walnut Brussels Sprouts

ingredients

2 cups of long-grain wild rice

2 tablespoons butter

3 tablespoons honey

1 cup minced Brussels sprouts

½ cup chopped walnuts

photo opposite

directions

1. Prepare the rice according to the package directions.
2. Melt the butter in a large skillet over medium heat. Add honey, Brussels sprouts, and walnuts.
3. Cook for 2 to 3 minutes.
4. Add the rice and toss. Cook for 1 to 2 minutes more.
5. Remove from heat.
6. Serve warm.

Rutabaga Bake

ingredients

1½ lbs of bacon

3 cups diced leeks

10 cups puréed rutabaga

2 sticks of butter at room temperature

½ cup heavy cream

¾ cup honey

1 teaspoon salt

1 teaspoon freshly ground pepper

2 garlic cloves, crushed

directions

1. Cook the bacon in a medium skillet until crisp. Set on a paper towel to remove excess grease.
2. When cool, chop or crumble.
3. Return the skillet to heat and add the leeks. Sauté until tender.
4. Preheat oven to 350°F.
5. In a large bowl, add puréed rutabagas, leeks, butter, cream, honey, garlic, salt, and pepper. Mix to combine.
6. Transfer into a baking dish and sprinkle the bacon on top.
7. Bake for 1 hour.
8. Serve warm.

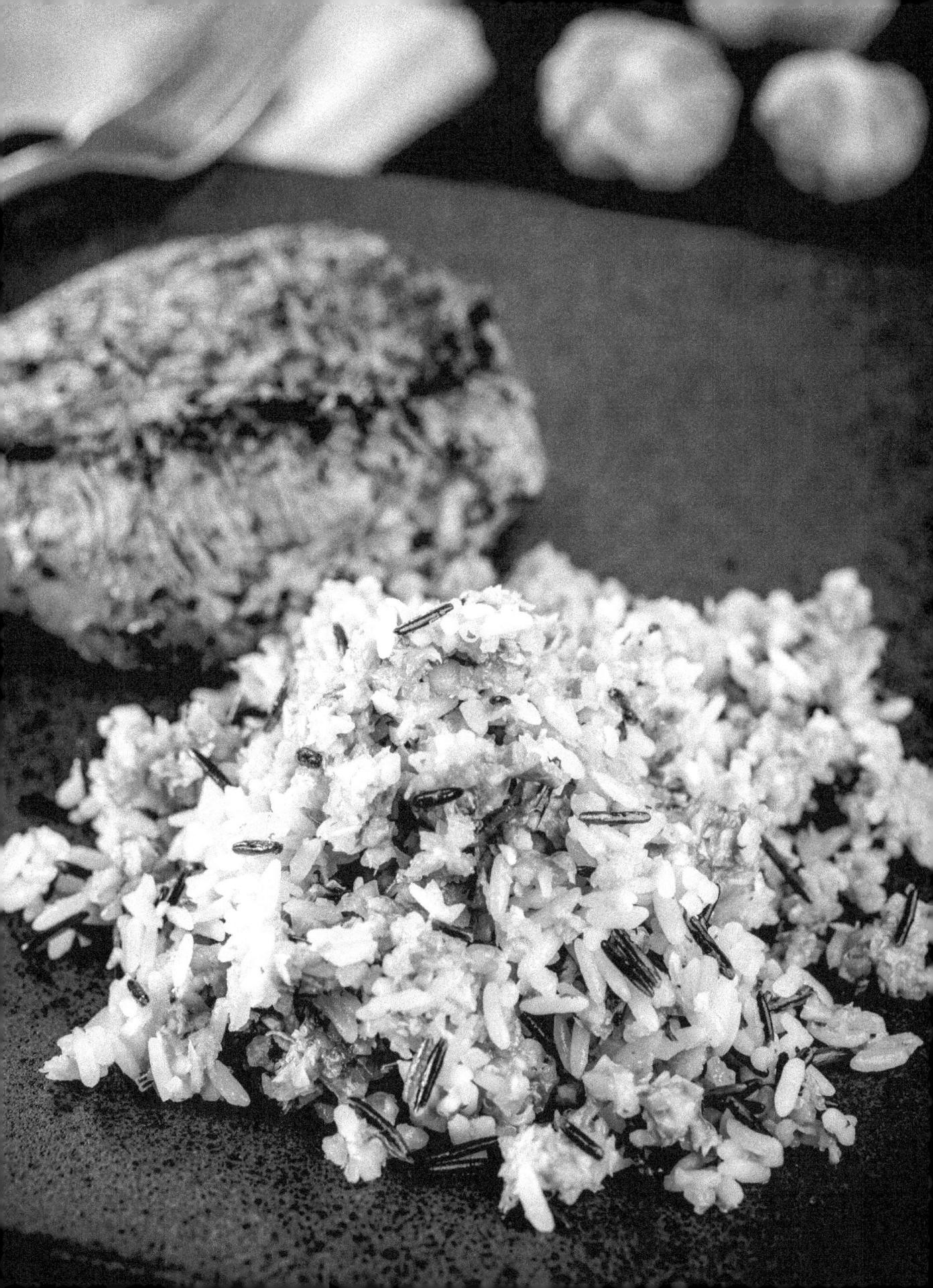

Sausage Broccoli Macaroni & Cheese

ingredients

1 lb. elbow macaroni

½ cup (8 tablespoons) unsalted butter, divided

½ cup flour

3 cups whole milk, room temperature

1 cup heavy cream, room temperature

4 cups grated Swiss cheese

2 cups grated sharp cheddar cheese

1 tablespoon chili powder

Coarse salt

Fresh ground pepper

1½ lbs. of fully cooked smoked sausage

1 cup riced broccoli

1 cup breadcrumbs

directions

1. Preheat the oven to 375°F.

2. Slice the smoked sausage into ½-inch sections. Set aside.

3. Cook the pasta according to the package directions. Drain, rinse with cool water, and spoon into a large bowl. Set aside.

4. Melt 6 tablespoons of the butter in a large pot over medium heat.

5. Add the flour and whisk continuously for 30 seconds or until fully blended.

6. Slowly add the milk and cream, whisking constantly until fully combined and smooth.

7. Reduce the heat to low.

8. Gradually add the shredded cheeses, stirring to combine completely. Add salt, pepper, and chili powder.

9. Remove from heat.

10. Pour cheese sauce over the prepared pasta. Add the riced broccoli and stir to blend.

11. Add the sausage and stir to coat completely with cheese sauce.

12. Pour into the prepared baking dish.

13. Melt the remaining 2 tablespoons of butter. Place the breadcrumbs in a small bowl, pour melted butter over them, and mix to create a crumb topping. Sprinkle on top of the pasta dish.

14. Bake for 30 to 40 minutes, until the breadcrumbs are golden brown and the cheese is bubbly.

15. Serve immediately.

Kohlrabi and Zucchini Fritters

directions

1. In a small saucepan, combine all the ingredients for the dipping sauce.

2. Cook on medium heat, stirring with a wooden spoon until the sugar dissolves.

3. Increase the heat to medium-high and allow to boil for 5 to 10 minutes, until the mixture thickens. Remove from heat and set aside. The sauce will continue to thicken as it cools.

4. Set the **zucchini** in a colander in the sink for 5 minutes, then press with your hands to ensure all excess water is removed.

5. In a large bowl, mix egg with salt, garlic powder, and chili powder. Add **minced kohlrabi** and **shredded zucchini**.

6. Mix with a spoon until fully blended.

7. In a deep pan or fryer, add 2 to 3 inches of vegetable oil. Heat it to 375°F, checking with a thermometer.

8. Form the batter into 3-inch to 4-inch round fritters. Cook up to three fritters at a time.

9. Fry each fritter until it is golden brown on one side, then flip and cook until the other side is golden brown too.

10. Once done, place the fritters on a plate lined with a paper towel to soak up the extra oil.

11. Serve warm as a side dish with the tangy dipping sauce.

ingredients: dipping sauce

¾ cup rice vinegar

½ cup sugar

1½ teaspoons red chili pepper flakes

1½ teaspoons salt

1 large garlic clove, minced

ingredients: fritters

1 egg

¼ teaspoon salt

¼ teaspoon garlic powder

¼ teaspoon chili powder

½ cup **minced kohlrabi**

1 cup **shredded zucchini**

vegetable oil for frying

Fiesta Corn

ingredients

1½ tablespoons butter

1 tablespoon chili powder

1 tablespoon cumin

½ teaspoon salt

½ teaspoon cilantro

4 cups of whole kernel corn

1 large diced jalapeño, seeds removed

1 cup **minced red bell pepper**

1 cup **minced green bell pepper**

⅔ cup diced onion

directions

1. Melt butter in a large saucepan over medium heat and add chili powder, cumin, salt, and cilantro. Whisk to blend until smooth without lumps.

2. Add corn, jalapeño, **red peppers,** green peppers, and onion. Stir to cover completely with sauce.

3. Cook for 5–7 minutes on medium-low heat, stirring frequently.

4. Serve warm.

Don't like the chunks? Try this saucy corn version:

1. Melt the butter.

2. Add the melted butter and all other ingredients except the corn into a food processor and set to high/purée. Pulse until the vegetables blend into the sauce.

3. Place the corn in a medium saucepan.
   *If using canned corn, drain to remove all liquid.

4. Add the blended sauce and stir.

5. Cook for 5 to 7 minutes on medium-low heat, stirring occasionally.

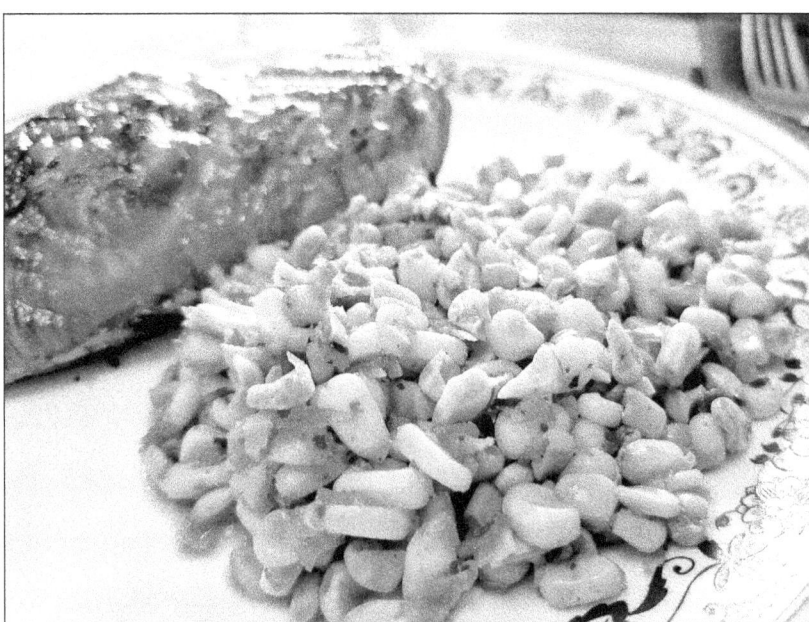

Grilled Vegetables

directions

1. Preheat an outdoor grill to 350°F.
2. Place all the prepared vegetable chunks in a large bowl. Set aside.
3. In a small bowl, mix olive oil, rosemary, minced garlic, seasoned salt, and pepper. Whisk to blend. Pour over the prepared vegetables.
4. Toss to coat the vegetables completely.
5. Lay out rectangular sheets of foil about 12-inches by 14 inches.
6. Place a portion of the vegetables in a single layer on one half of the foil, then fold and secure all the edges.
7. Repeat until all the vegetables have been secured in foil packs.
8. Place on the grill for 25 to 30 minutes or until the veggies are tender.
9. Remove from grill. Top with Creamy Pepper Kale Mayo (p. 60).
10. Serve immediately.

TIP: Put your homemade mayo in a squeeze bottle for easy serving!

ingredients

2 cups peeled butternut squash, chopped into ½-inch slices

1 rutabaga, peeled and chopped into 1-inch cubes

2 carrots, peeled and chopped into ½-inch slices

4 or 5 asparagus stalks, diced

¼ cup diced leeks or sweet onion

3 tablespoons olive oil

1 tablespoon chopped fresh rosemary or 1 teaspoon dried rosemary

2 garlic cloves, minced

2 teaspoons seasoned salt

1 teaspoon pepper

Creamy Pepper Kale Mayo (p. 60)

Sweet Potato Fries

ingredients

1 sweet potato

1 tablespoon seasoning salt

½ tablespoon pepper

directions

1. Preheat deep fryer to 350° F.
2. Wash sweet potato and pat dry.
3. Cut the potato longways in half, then again. Continue slicing until the potato is cut into roughly ½" match-stick like strips.
4. Cook in deep fryer for 8 minutes.
5. Remove and set on paper towels for 2 to 3 minutes.
6. Increase fryer temperature to 400° F.
7. Place sweet potato fries in the deep fryer again and cook an additional 4 minutes
8. Place on paper towel briefly to remove excess oil.
9. Put in large bowl and immediately toss in seasoning salt and pepper. Serve Hot.

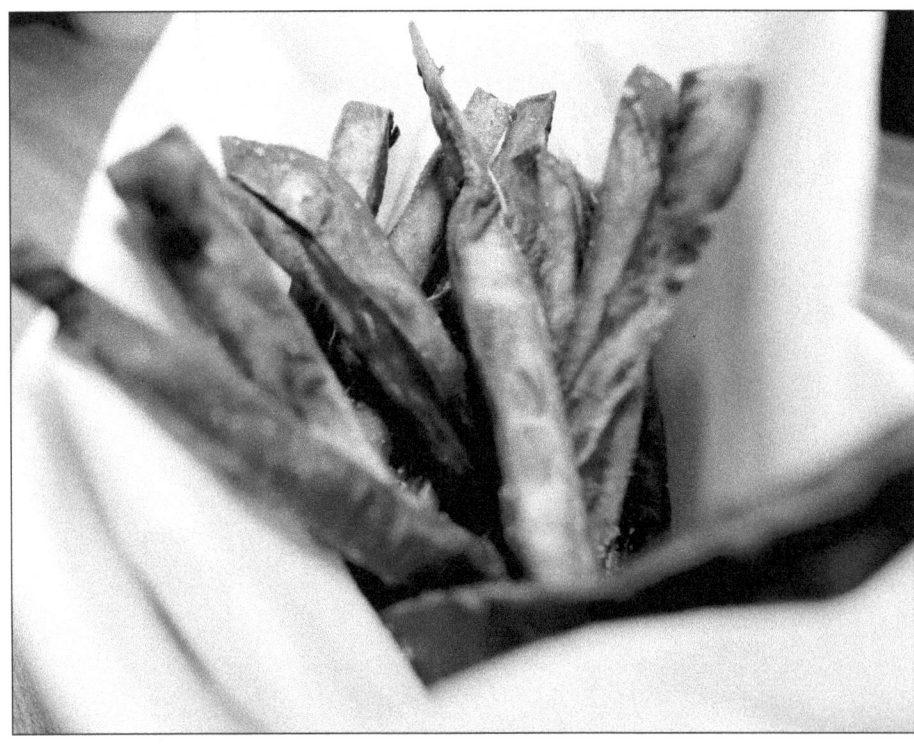

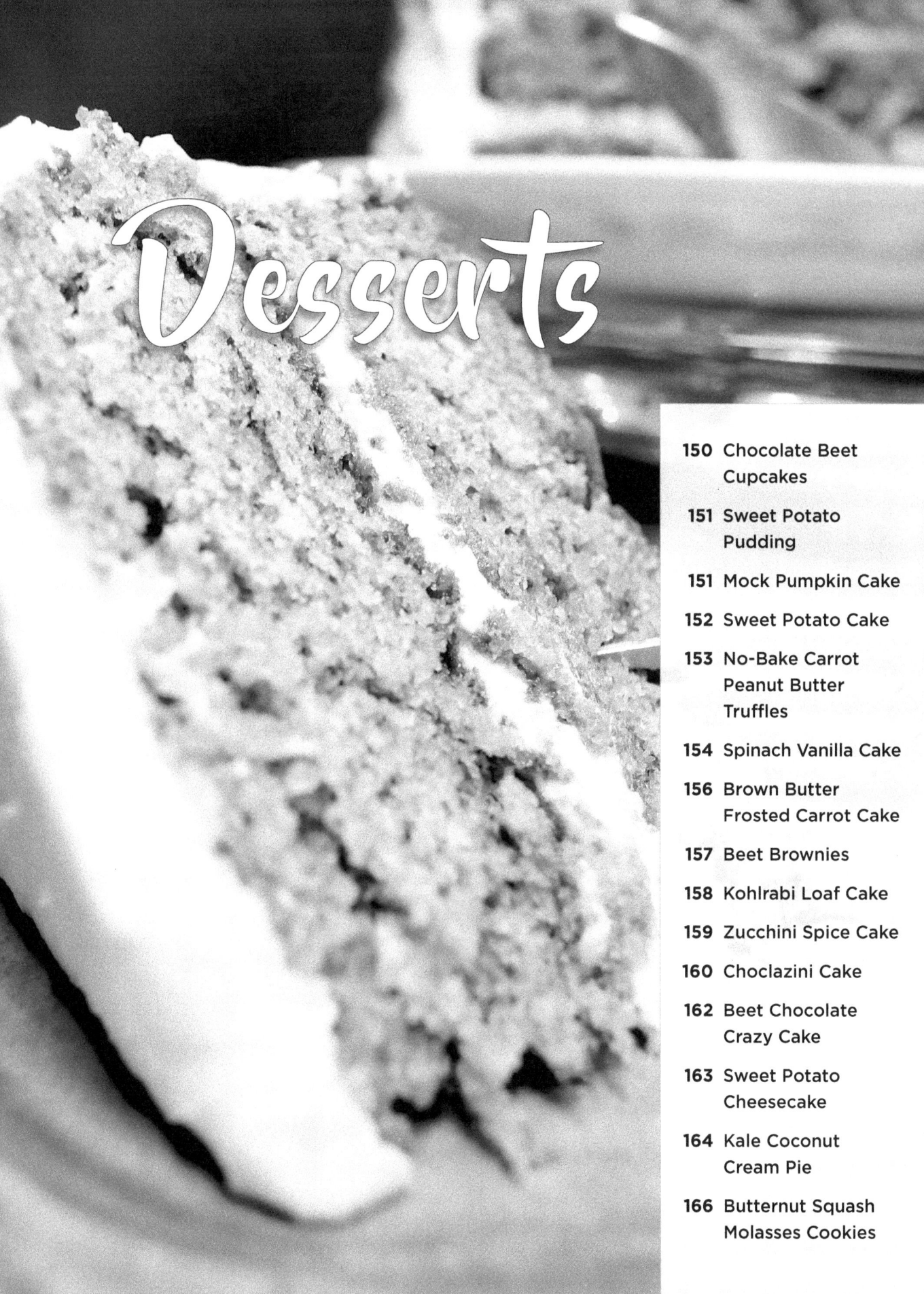

Desserts

150 Chocolate Beet Cupcakes

151 Sweet Potato Pudding

151 Mock Pumpkin Cake

152 Sweet Potato Cake

153 No-Bake Carrot Peanut Butter Truffles

154 Spinach Vanilla Cake

156 Brown Butter Frosted Carrot Cake

157 Beet Brownies

158 Kohlrabi Loaf Cake

159 Zucchini Spice Cake

160 Choclazini Cake

162 Beet Chocolate Crazy Cake

163 Sweet Potato Cheesecake

164 Kale Coconut Cream Pie

166 Butternut Squash Molasses Cookies

Chocolate Beet Cupcakes

ingredients

½ cup unsweetened natural cocoa powder

¾ cup all-purpose flour

½ teaspoon baking soda

¾ teaspoon baking powder

¼ teaspoon salt

2 eggs at room temperature

½ cup granulated sugar

½ cup packed light brown sugar

⅓ cup **puréed beets**

2 teaspoons vanilla extract

1 teaspoon cream of tartar

½ cup buttermilk

directions

1. Preheat the oven to 350°F.

2. Line a 12-cup muffin pan with cupcake liners.

3. In a large bowl, whisk the cocoa powder, flour, baking soda, baking powder, and salt until thoroughly combined. Set aside.

4. In a medium bowl, whisk the eggs, granulated sugar, brown sugar, **puréed beets,** and vanilla together until completely smooth.

5. Gradually spoon the wet ingredients (medium bowl) into the dry ingredients (large bowl). Blend until fully mixed.

6. Slowly add the buttermilk and mix slightly until just combined; do not overmix.

7. Pour this batter into the liners. Only fill about ¾ because the batter will expand during baking.

8. Bake in batches for 18 to 20 minutes, or until a toothpick inserted in the center comes out clean.

9. Allow to cool completely before frosting.

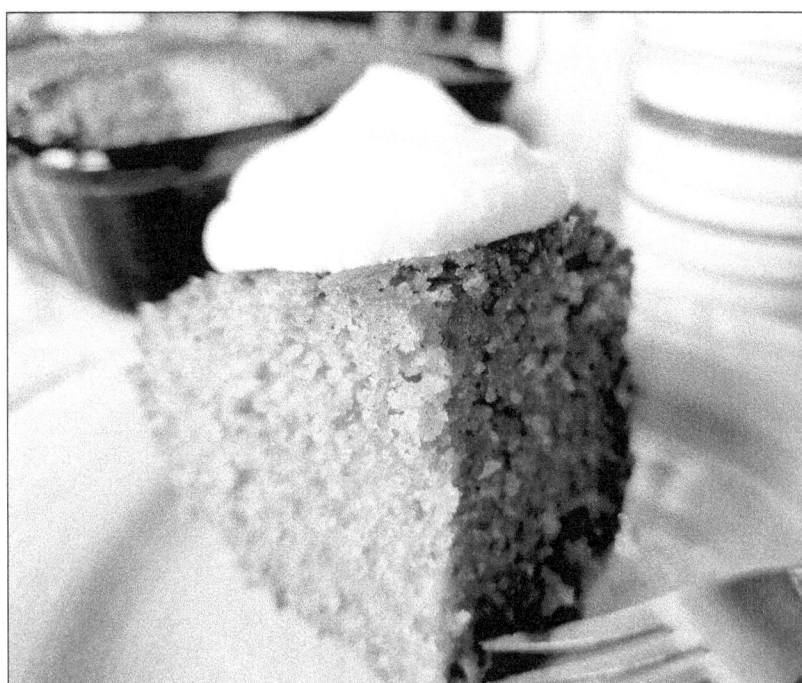

Mock Pumpkin Cake recipe opposite page.

Sweet Potato Pudding

directions

1. Preheat oven to 325°F.
2. Spray an 8-inch square baking dish with non-stick spray. Set aside.
3. In a large bowl, combine the sweet potato purée with all the remaining ingredients.
4. Mix well to blend.
5. Pour into the prepared baking dish.
6. Bake for 60 minutes.
7. Cool on a wire rack.
8. Serve with whipped topping.

ingredients

4 cups puréed sweet potato

1 stick unsalted butter; room temperature

¾ cup brown sugar

One 12-ounce can of evaporated milk

3 eggs

1 tablespoon cinnamon

½ fresh nutmeg, grated

¼ teaspoon salt

¼ teaspoon ginger

Whipped topping

Mock Pumpkin Cake

directions

1. Preheat oven to 350°F.
2. Spray an 8-inch square cake pan with non-stick cooking oil. Set aside.
3. Add all the ingredients to a large bowl.
4. Using a hand mixer on low, blend until combined.
5. Pour into the prepared pan.
6. Bake for 45 minutes.
7. Cool completely.
8. Slice into squares for serving.

NOTE: Use a bread pan to make a snack cake. It's even better topped with your favorite frosting or whipped topping as shown opposite page).

ingredients

2 cups butternut squash purée

4 eggs

½ cup water

½ cup canola oil

1⅔ cups sugar

2 cups flour

2 teaspoons baking powder

1 teaspoon baking soda

1 teaspoon salt

1 teaspoon cinnamon

1¼ teaspoons nutmeg

Sweet Potato Cake

ingredients

4 eggs

½ cup water

½ cup oil

1⅔ cups sugar

2 cups flour

2 teaspoons baking powder

1 teaspoon baking soda

1 teaspoon salt

1 teaspoon cinnamon

1¼ teaspoons nutmeg

2 cups puréed sweet potato

4 tablespoons unsalted butter, diced

2 tablespoons brown sugar

cream cheese frosting

8 oz. cream cheese, at room temperature

4 tablespoons unsalted butter, at room temperature

1 teaspoon vanilla extract

2 cups powdered sugar

directions

1. Preheat oven to 350° F.

2. Spray a 9-inch square cake pan with non-stick cooking spray. Set aside.

3. Whisk the eggs, water, and oil in a large bowl to blend. Add puréed sweet potato, butter, and brown sugar.

4. In a separate bowl, sift together sugar, flour, baking powder, baking soda, salt, cinnamon, and nutmeg.

5. Pour the sweet potato mixture into the flour mixture and stir well to blend.

6. Pour into the prepared pan.

7. Bake for 45 minutes, or until toothpick comes out clean. Remove from oven and cool on wire rack.

8. While cake is cooling, prepare the frosting. In a medium-size bowl, beat the cream cheese and butter until completely smooth. Add the vanilla and ½ cup of the powdered sugar, beating slowly until smooth. Gradually add remaining powdered sugar and beat until smooth.

9. Top the cake with prepared cream cheese frosting when cooled.

No-Bake Carrot Peanut Butter Truffles

directions

1. In a medium bowl, add all the ingredients except the ground nuts.
2. Mix well until combined.
3. Form into balls and roll in the ground nuts until covered.
4. Place on a parchment-lined tray.
5. Store in refrigerator.

ingredients

½ cup riced carrot

¼ cup puffed rice

3 tablespoons peanut butter

1 teaspoon honey

½ teaspoon ground cinnamon

⅛ teaspoon ground ginger

¼ cup ground walnuts or pecans

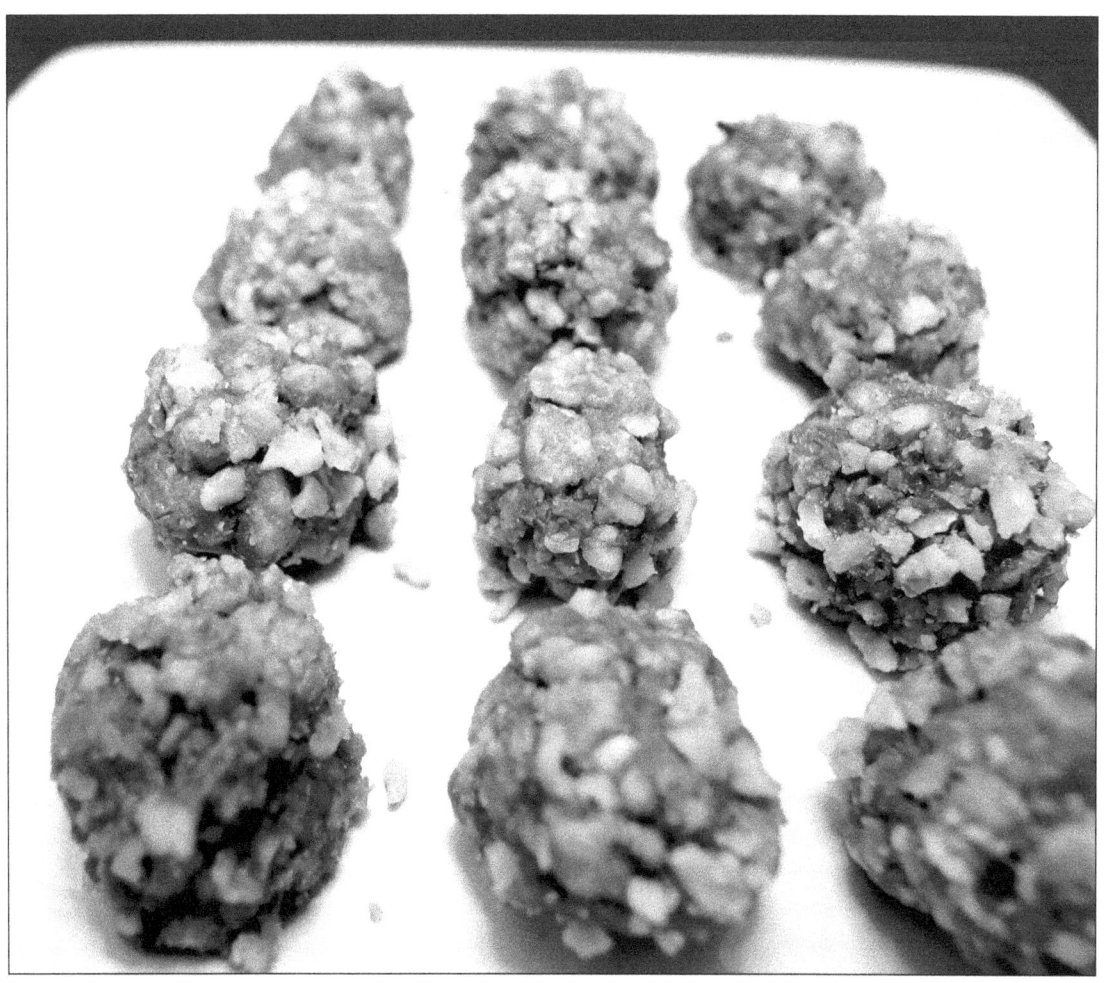

Desserts

Spinach Vanilla Cake

ingredients: cake

3 eggs

2 teaspoons vanilla extract

⅔ cup brown sugar

⅔ cup honey

½ cup melted butter, cooled

1½ cups **spinach purée**

2 cups all-purpose flour

3 teaspoons baking powder

½ teaspoon baking soda

½ teaspoon salt

ingredients: frosting

2 cups unsalted butter at room temperature

½ teaspoon salt

6 cups powdered sugar

5–6 tablespoons heavy cream

1 tablespoon light corn syrup

2 teaspoons vanilla extract

directions

1. Preheat oven to 350° F.

2. Spray two 8-inch round cake pans with non-stick cooking oil and dust with flour.

3. In a large bowl, mix together eggs, vanilla, brown sugar, honey, and butter. Add **puréed spinach** and stir until combined.

4. Sift together the flour, baking powder, baking soda, and salt. Add this mix to the wet ingredients and stir to combine.

5. Divide the batter between the two prepared cake pans.

6. Bake for 25 minutes or until a toothpick inserted into the center comes out clean.

7. Cool for 5 minutes in the pans and then place on a wire rack to cool completely.

8. While the cakes are cooling, prepare the frosting.

9. Beat the butter with an electric mixer until creamy. Add salt and vanilla extract and blend.

10. Gradually add powdered sugar, ½ cup at a time, and slowly mix until 3 cups have been mixed.

11. Add the heavy cream and corn syrup, then gradually add the remaining powdered sugar.

12. Add more cream as needed to achieve the desired consistency.

13. Place one layer of the cake on a serving plate or platform. Spread a layer of frosting. Top with a second layer of cake. Cover the top and sides completely with the frosting.

14. Slice and serve.

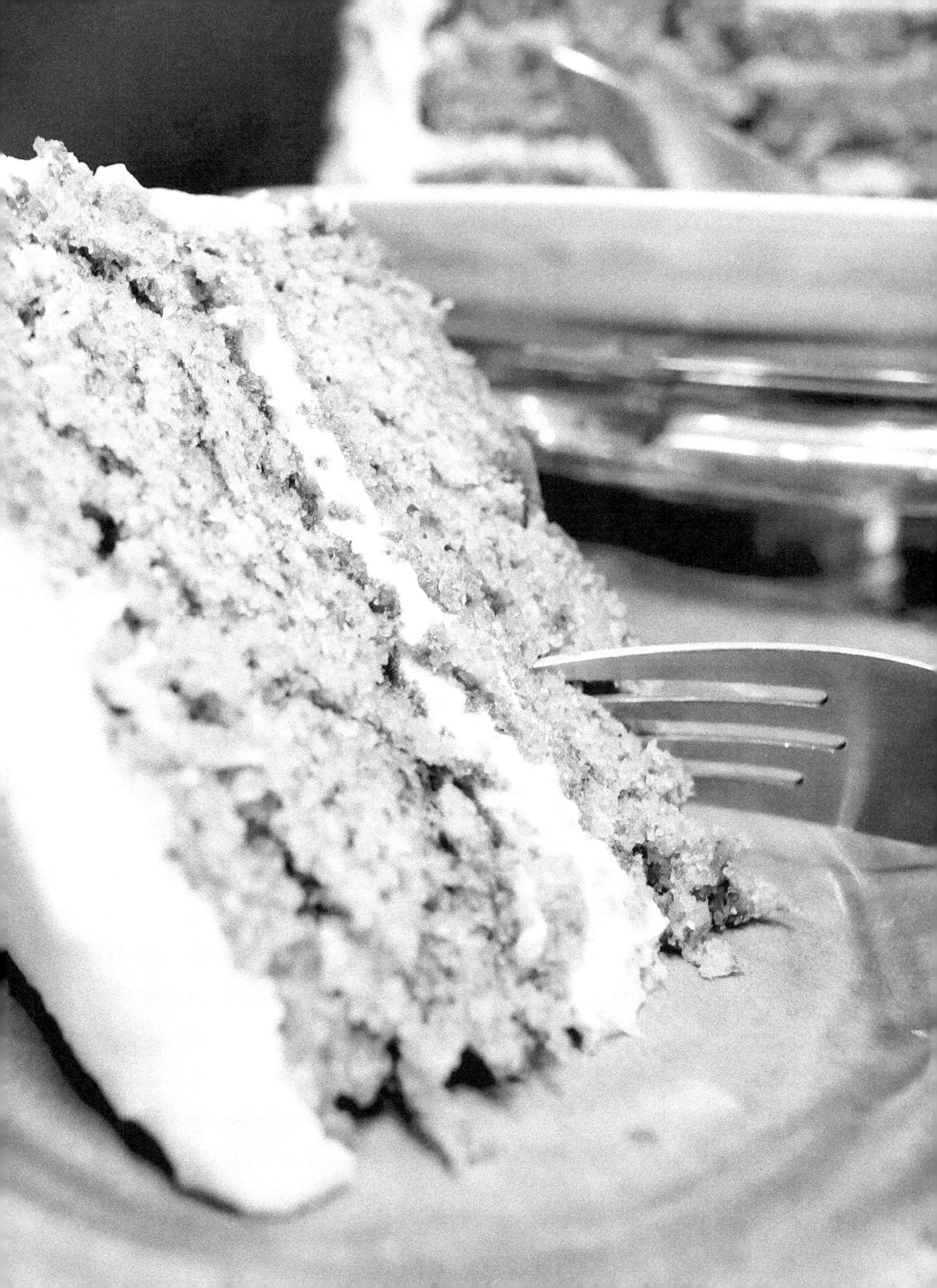

Brown Butter Frosted Carrot Cake

ingredients: cake

2 eggs

¼ cup canola oil

¼ cup melted butter

2 tablespoons honey

2 teaspoons vanilla extract

½ cup packed light brown sugar (or substitute unsweetened applesauce)

1¼ cups all-purpose flour

1 teaspoon baking powder

½ teaspoon baking soda

½ teaspoon salt

2 teaspoons ground cinnamon

½ teaspoon ground nutmeg

½ teaspoon ground cardamom

2 cups packed riced carrots

ingredients: frosting

½ cup butter

4 cups powdered sugar

1½ teaspoons vanilla extract

3 tablespoons milk

directions

1. Preheat the oven to 350°F.

2. Spray an 8-inch square cake pan with non-stick cooking oil. Set aside.

3. In a large bowl, add eggs, oil, melted butter, honey, vanilla, and brown sugar or applesauce. Slowly blend by hand or electric mixer on low speed until smooth.

4. In a medium bowl, whisk flour, baking powder, baking soda, salt, cinnamon, nutmeg, and cardamom.

5. Slowly add the dry ingredients by hand to the wet ingredients. Mix lightly with a rubber spatula or spoon just until blended. Do not overmix.

6. Fold in the carrots.

7. Spoon the batter into the prepared pan.

8. Bake for 30 to 40 minutes or until a tester poked into the center of the cake comes out clean or with a few moist crumbs attached. Set the cake aside to cool.

9. While the cake cools, make the frosting by heating butter in a large saucepan over medium heat until boiling.

10. When the butter turns a delicate brown, remove it from heat immediately.

11. Add the powdered sugar, vanilla extract, and milk. Whisk together until smooth.

12. Using a spatula, spread the brown butter frosting over the warm cake.

Beet Brownies

directions

1. Preheat oven to 325°F.
2. Spray a 9-inch square cake pan with non-stick cooking oil. Set aside.
3. In a medium bowl, cream the butter and honey together.
4. Add the **puréed beets,** vanilla, and eggs. Mix well.
5. In a separate bowl, whisk together the cocoa powder, flour, and baking soda.
6. Add the dry ingredients to the wet and stir until combined.
7. Stir in the chocolate chips.
8. Pour the batter into the prepared baking pan.
9. Bake for about 35 to 40 minutes or until a toothpick inserted into the center comes out clean.
10. Set on a wire rack to cool.
11. Cut into squares and serve.

ingredients

½ cup butter

½ cup honey

1 cup **puréed beets**

1 teaspoon vanilla

2 eggs

½ cup cocoa powder

½ cup flour

¼ teaspoon baking soda

¾ cup milk chocolate chips

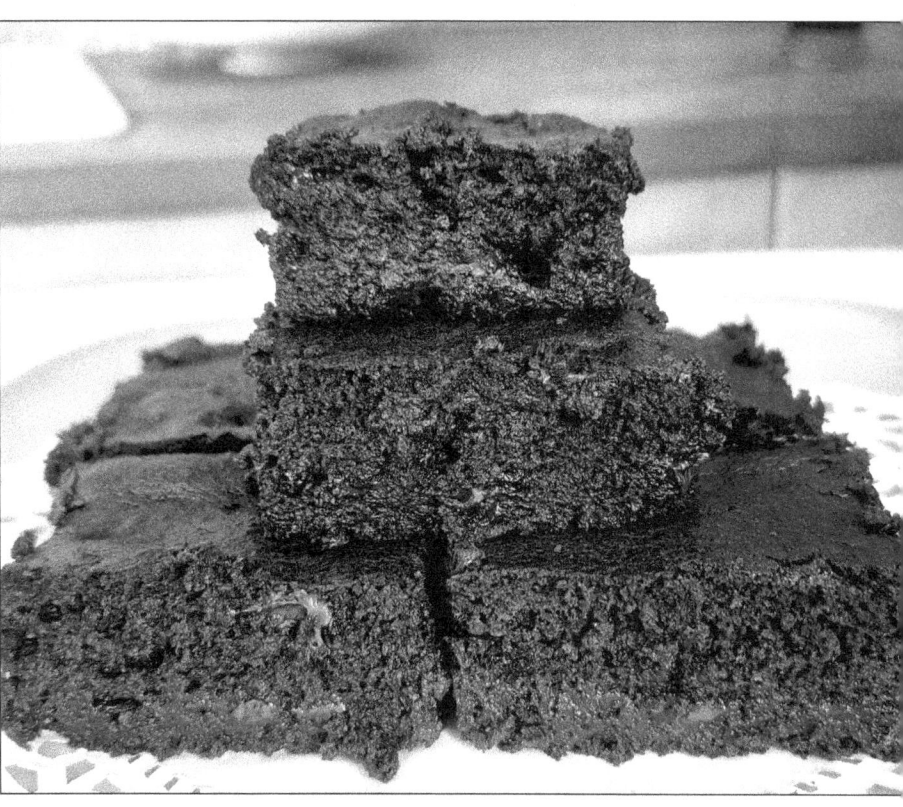

Kohlrabi Loaf Cake

ingredients: cake

¾ cup unsalted butter at room temperature

¾ cup sugar

3 eggs

1⅔ cups all-purpose flour

2 teaspoons baking powder

3 tablespoons milk

1 teaspoon nutmeg

1 cup **minced kohlrabi**

ingredients: glaze

1 cup powdered sugar

½ teaspoon vanilla extract

½ teaspoon almond extract

½ teaspoon cornstarch

2 tablespoons milk

directions

1. Preheat the oven to 350°F.

2. Spray a 9x5 loaf pan with non-stick cooking spray.

3. In a large bowl, cream the butter and sugar until light and fluffy. And the eggs one at a time and beat each one in thoroughly.

4. Add the flour and baking powder, mixing well. Add the milk and nutmeg, stirring to combine.

5. Add **kohlrabi,** mixing well.

6. Pour the mixture into the prepared loaf pan and bake for 60 minutes or until a toothpick comes out clean.

7. Cool the cake in the pan for 15 minutes and then remove from the pan.

8. To prepare the glaze, add all the ingredients to a medium bowl. Whisk by hand or use a hand mixer to blend.

9. Drizzle glaze over the cake, allowing it to run down the sides.

10. Cool completely before slicing.

11. Store the loaf covered for up to four days. Freezes well.

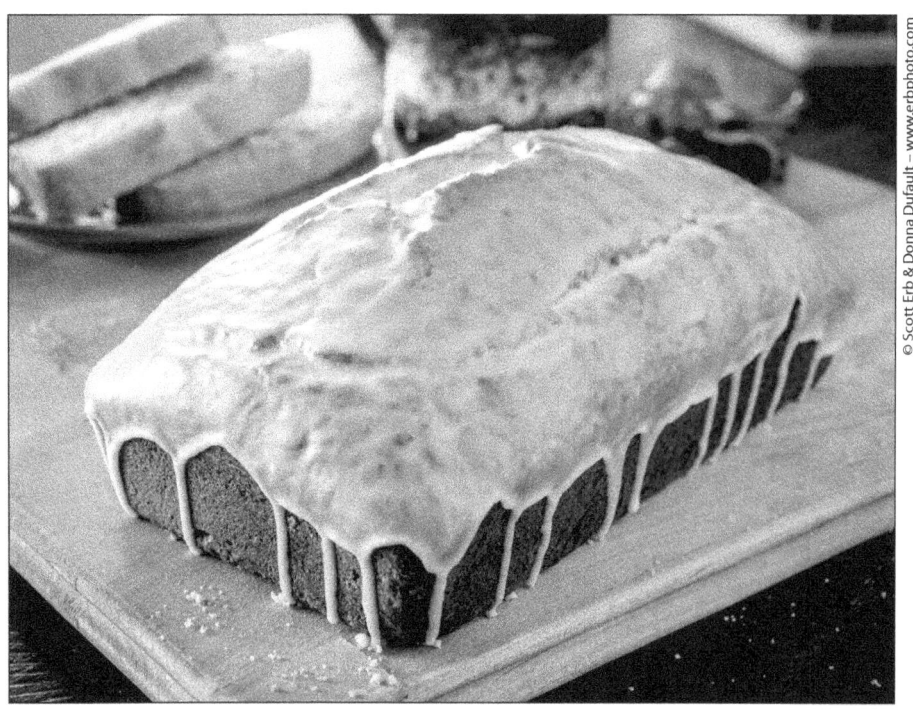

© Scott Erb & Donna Dufault – www.erbphoto.com

Zucchini Spice Cake

directions

1. Preheat oven to 350°F.
2. Spray two 8-inch round cake pans with non-stick cooking spray and dust with flour. If making cupcakes, fill two muffin tins with cupcake liners.
3. In a large bowl, mix the brown sugar, sour cream, eggs, canola oil, and vanilla extract.
4. Add in the flour, baking soda, baking powder, and spices. Mix until blended.
5. Fold in the **zucchini** and coconut.
6. Divide equally between the cake pans. For cupcakes, fill until ⅔ full.
7. Bake for 30 to 35 minutes, or until a toothpick inserted into the center comes out clean.
8. Cool on racks. Remove from the cake pans and cool completely.
9. For frosting, add all the ingredients into a medium bowl and blend with an electric mixer until smooth.
10. Place one layer of the cake on a serving plate or platform. Spread a layer of frosting. Top with a second layer of cake. Cover the top and sides completely with the frosting.
11. Slice and serve.

ingredients: cake

¾ cup brown sugar

⅓ cup sour cream

2 eggs

½ cup canola oil

2 teaspoons vanilla extract

1 cup flour

1 teaspoon baking soda

1 teaspoon baking powder

1 teaspoon cinnamon

1 teaspoon nutmeg

1 teaspoon ginger

½ teaspoon salt

¼ teaspoon pepper

⅔ cup **shredded zucchini**

⅓ cup flake coconut

ingredients: frosting

½ stick unsalted butter

2 cups powdered icing sugar

1 teaspoon vanilla extract

1 tablespoon milk

Choclazini Cake

ingredients: cake

3½ cups flour, all-purpose

¾ cup cocoa powder, unsweetened

¾ teaspoon salt

2 teaspoons baking soda

1 banana

⅓ cup butter, melted and cooled

1 cup sugar

½ cup honey

¼ cup packed brown sugar

3 large eggs

2 teaspoons vanilla extract

¾ cup sour cream

4 cups **shredded zucchini**, excess water removed

1 cup semi-sweet chocolate chips

ingredients: glaze

2 tablespoons sugar

½ cup heavy cream

4 ounce chopped semi-sweet chocolate

2 tablespoons corn syrup

Shaved chocolate or multicolored sprinkles (optional)

directions

1. Preheat oven to 350°F.

2. Spray a bundt pan with non-stick cooking oil and dust with cocoa powder.

3. In a medium bowl, combine flour, cocoa powder, salt, and baking soda. Set aside.

4. Mash a small peeled banana in a large bowl. Add butter, sugar, honey, brown sugar, eggs, vanilla, and sour cream.

5. Gradually mix in the dry ingredients, stirring until almost combined.

6. Add the **shredded zucchini** and the mini chocolate chips and stir lightly to mix. Do not over-blend.

7. Pour into the prepared bundt pan and bake for 60 to 75 minutes or until an inserted knife or toothpick comes out clean.

chocolate glaze

1. Heat the heavy cream and sugar in a small saucepan over medium heat until the sugar is dissolved.

2. Put the chocolate and corn syrup in a medium-sized bowl and pour the heated mixture over it.

3. Wait 1 to 2 minutes for the heat to melt the chocolate, then whisk until smooth.

4. Cool for 5 minutes, then drizzle over the top of the cake.

5. Top with shaved chocolate or sprinkles.

6. Slice and serve.

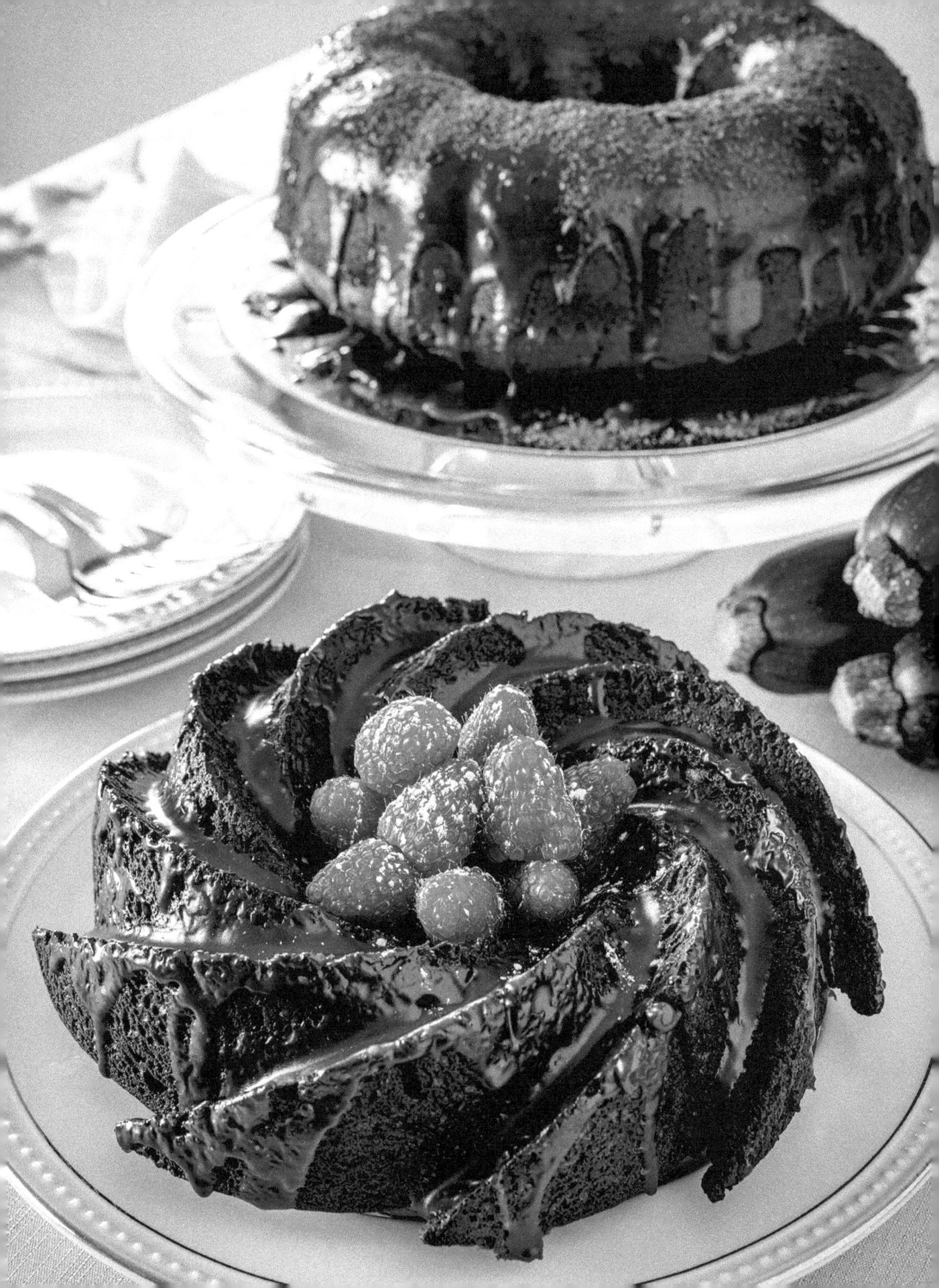

Beet Chocolate Crazy Cake

ingredients

1½ cups flour

3 tablespoons unsweetened cocoa

1 cup sugar

1 teaspoon baking soda

½ teaspoon salt

⅓ cup **puréed beets**

1 teaspoon apple cider vinegar

1 teaspoon pure vanilla extract

1 cup black coffee (cooled)

directions

1. Preheat oven to 350°F.

2. Spray a 9-inch square cake pan with non-stick cooking oil. Set aside.

3. In a medium bowl, combine flour, cocoa, sugar, baking soda, and salt.

4. Add **puréed beets** and apple cider vinegar, mixing to blend.

5. Add coffee and vanilla. Mix until smooth.

6. Pour into the prepared baking pan.

7. Bake on the middle rack of the oven for 35 minutes. Check with a toothpick to make sure it comes out clean.

8. Place on a wire rack to cool. Top with your favorite frosting when cooled.

9. Slice and serve.

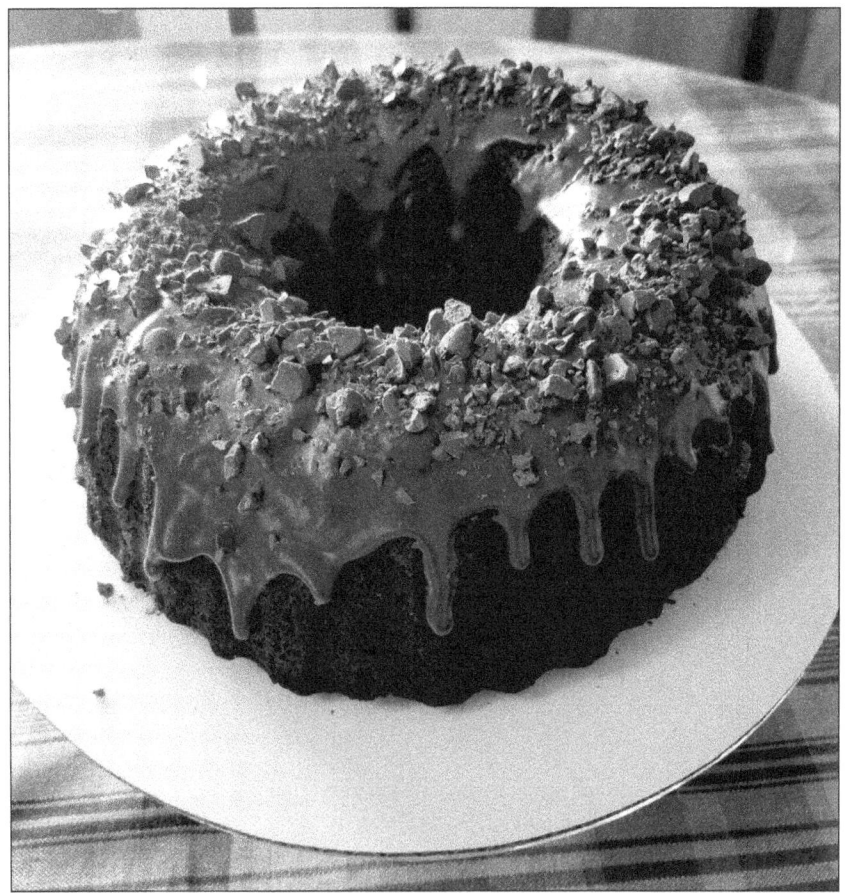

Photo shows cake frosted and sprinkled with chopped milk chocolate chips.

Sweet Potato Cheesecake

directions

1. Preheat oven to 350°F.
2. In a medium bowl, combine the graham cracker crumbs, pecans, and sugar. Pour in the melted butter and blend with a fork until moistened.
3. Press the mixture firmly into the bottom of a 9-inch springform pan. Bake for 8 to 10 minutes, then remove from the oven and set on a wire rack to cool.

filling

1. In a large bowl, beat cream cheese, molasses, and brown sugar until smooth.
2. Add eggs one at a time, mixing well after each addition.
3. In a separate bowl, whisk together the cornstarch, cinnamon, nutmeg, and ginger.
4. Add to the cream cheese mixture and mix.
5. Add the sweet potato purée, sour cream, water, and vanilla. Mix until fully combined and creamy.
6. Pour into the prepared and cooled crust.
7. Place the springform pan in a larger baking pan.
8. Fill the larger pan with hot water until it reaches halfway up the sides of the springform pan.
9. Bake for 60 to 70 minutes, or until the center of the batter is set but slightly jiggly.
10. Turn off the oven, crack the door, and let the cheesecake cool in the oven for 1 hour.
11. Remove and refrigerate for at least 4 hours or overnight.
12. Slice and serve. Refrigerate leftovers.

ingredients: crust

1½ cups graham cracker crumbs

⅓ cup ground pecans

¼ cup sugar

3 tablespoons melted butter

ingredients: filling

8 ounces cream cheese, softened

½ cup molasses

½ cup brown sugar

2 eggs

2 tablespoons cornstarch

½ teaspoon ground cinnamon

¼ teaspoon ground nutmeg

¼ teaspoon ginger

1¾ cups sweet potato purée

¾ cup of sour cream or plain yogurt

¼ cup of water

1 teaspoon vanilla

Kale Coconut Cream Pie

ingredients

One 9-inch premade pie crust

2½ cups whole milk, divided

¾ cup shredded coconut

4 tablespoons cornstarch

½ cup granulated sugar

⅛ teaspoon salt

2 eggs

2 teaspoons vanilla extract

2 cups **puréed kale**

2 cups whipped topping

directions

1. Preheat the oven to 350°F.

2. Place the crust in a pie pan. Use a fork to prick the crust to allow air to escape. This will keep the crust flat as it bakes.

3. Bake for 18 to 20 minutes, or until it just starts to turn golden.

4. Remove from the oven and cool.

5. In a small bowl, add a ½ cup of milk to the ¾ cup of coconut and set aside to soak.

6. Whisk the sugar, cornstarch, and salt in a medium saucepan.

7. Place over medium heat. Add eggs, vanilla, and **puréed kale.**

8. Whisk in the remaining 2 cups of milk and the soaked shredded coconut. Whisk continuously for 5 to 7 minutes until thickened.

9. Remove from heat and stir to cool. Pour the filling into a bowl and allow to cool completely to room temperature. When cool, chill in the refrigerator for an hour.

10. Remove from refrigerator and spoon into the cooled pie crust. Chill for another 2–3 hours.

11. Top with the whipped topping.

12. Slice and serve.

13. Store the leftovers in the refrigerator.

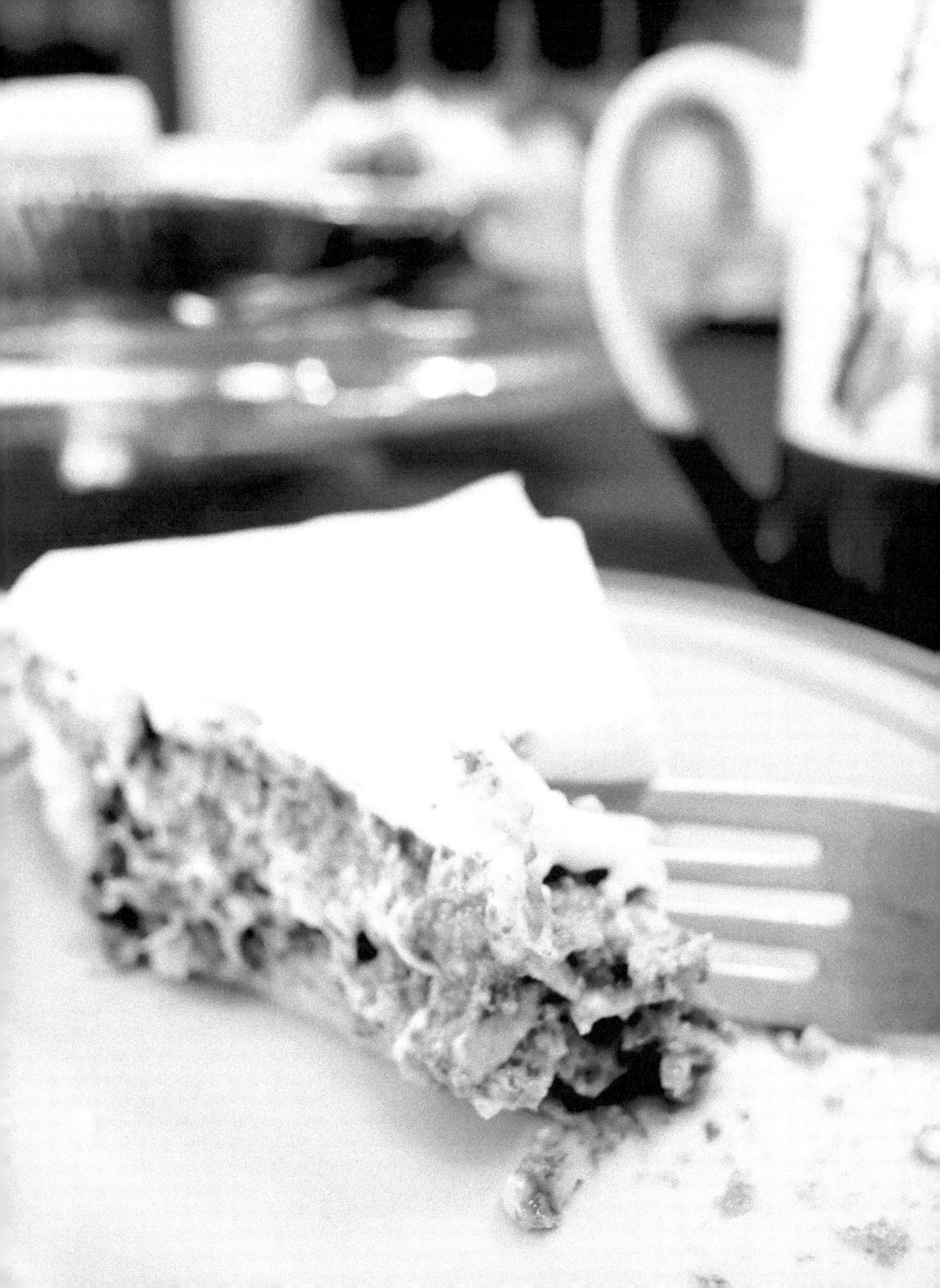

Butternut Squash Molasses Cookies

ingredients

1⅓ cups all-purpose flour

2 cups old-fashioned oats

½ teaspoon baking powder

½ teaspoon baking soda

½ cup unsalted butter, softened

¼ cup brown sugar

¼ cup granulated sugar

2 tablespoons molasses

1 egg

1 teaspoon vanilla extract

1 teaspoon ground cinnamon

1 teaspoon ground ginger

¼ teaspoon ground cloves

3 cups butternut squash purée

ingredients: frosting

½ cup (1 stick) salted butter

4 cups confectioners' sugar

1 teaspoon vanilla extract

¼ to ⅓ cup milk

¼ cup ground pecans (optional)

directions

1. Preheat the oven to 350°F.

2. Line a baking tray with parchment paper.

3. In a large bowl, whisk the flour, oats, baking powder, and baking soda. Set aside.

4. In a medium bowl, cream together the butter and both sugars. Mix until light and fluffy.

5. Add the molasses, egg, vanilla, and spices. Mix well.

6. Fold in the puréed butternut squash. Add the dry ingredients to the batter and stir until combined.

7. Drop teaspoonfuls of the mixture onto the prepared baking tray.

8. Bake for 8 to 10 minutes or until golden.

9. Allow to cool for 2 to 3 minutes on the tray and then transfer to a wire rack to cool completely.

10. While cookies are cooling, prepare frosting.

11. In a large saucepan, heat butter over medium heat. It is best to have a thin layer of butter in the pan so that it heats evenly. Allow butter to heat until boiling. Watching constantly, allow butter turn a delicate brown and remove from heat immediately.

12. Add powdered sugar, vanilla extract, and milk into the saucepan, whisking until smooth.

13. Spread the brown butter frosting on cookies while frosting is still warm. It will set up and not spread well when cooled.

14. Sprinkle with ground pecans if using.

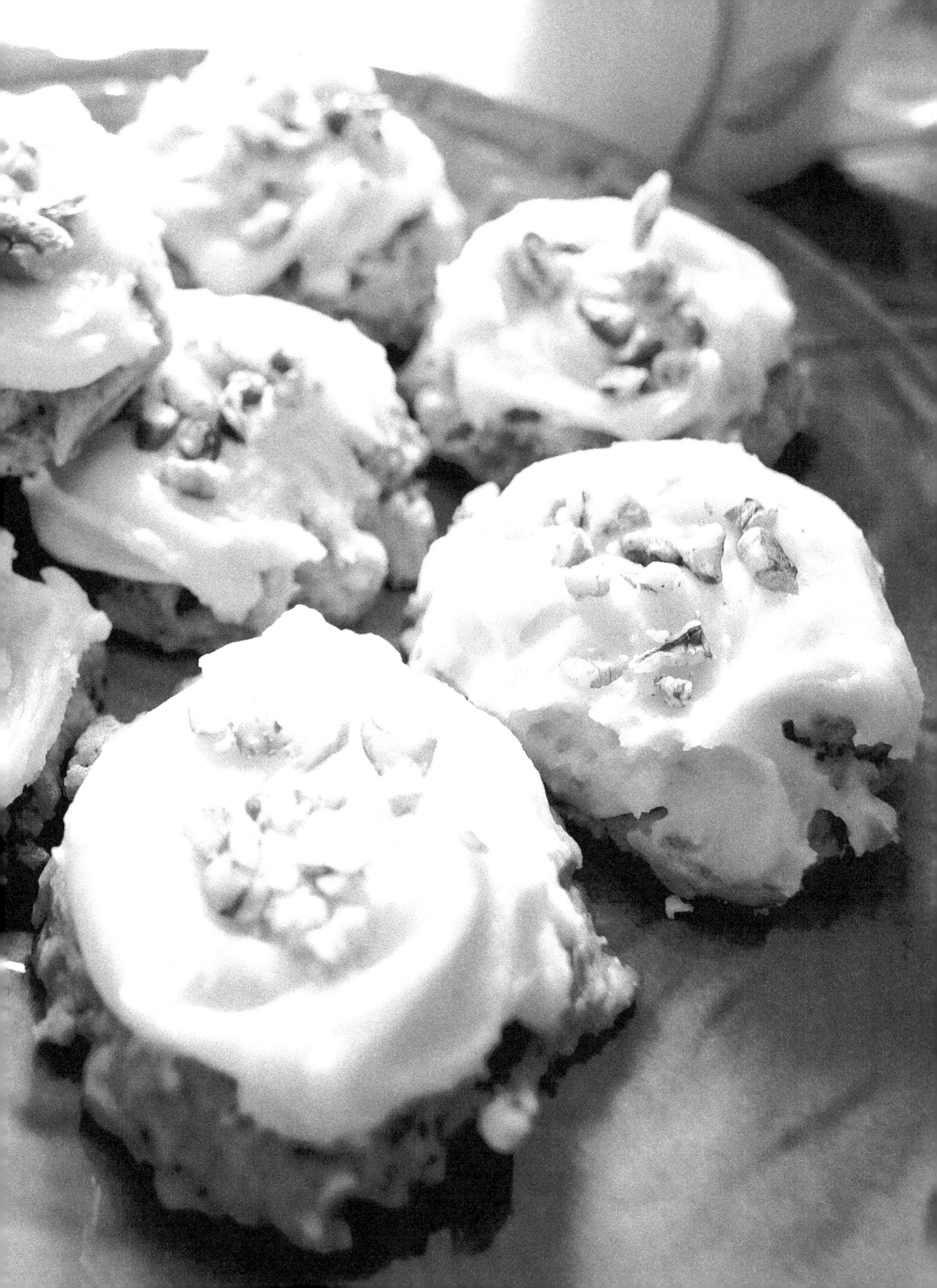

Index

Asparagus
Buying & Storing 8
Chopped & Purée 43
Asparagus Frittata 94
Chicken Tetrazzini with Asparagus 126
Cauliflower au Gratin Pasta 137
Grilled Vegetables 147

Beets
Buying & Storing 9
Roasted 26
Purée 27
Juice 28
Beef Bourguignon 108
Beet Brownies 157
Beet Chocolate Crazy Cake 162
Beet Hummus 62
Chocolate Beet Cupcakes 150
Crockpot Pasta Bolognese-style Sauce 130
Fresh Veggie Noodles 118
Fruity Beetroot Jelly 56
Glazed Beet Donuts 102
Sweet & Savory Squash &
   Root Veggies 141

Bell Pepper
Buying & Storing 9
Purée 29
Minced 30
Crockpot Breakfast Casserole 101
Fiesta Corn 146
Omelet Muffins 106
Shepherd's Pie 124
Smooth Salsa 61
Spicy Pumpkin Bread 85
Stuffed Pasta Shells 129
Veggie Crust Mini Pizza 71
Veggie Peanut Chicken
   & Zucchini Noodles 122

Broccoli
Buying & Storing 10
Riced & Minced 44
Broccoli Bread 78
Buffalo Broccoli Cheese Sauce 59
Easy Vegetable Soup 74
Nutty Egg Waffles 97
Potato Broccoli Soup 73
Sausage Broccoli Macaroni & Cheese 144
Savory Mini Meat Pies 66
Tangy Meatballs 72
Veggie Poppers 70

Brussels Sprouts
Buying & Storing 10
Minced 45
Beef Hotpot 117
Cowboy Beans 140
Easy Vegetable Soup 74
Honey Walnut Brussels Sprouts 142
Nutty Egg Waffles 97
Veggie Peanut Chicken
   & Zucchini Noodles 122

Butternut Squash
Buying & Storing 11
Purée 37
Butternut Squash Cornbread 79
Butternut Squash Molasses Cookies 166
Grilled Vegetables 147
Mock Pumpkin Cake 151
Sweet & Savory Squash & Root Veggies 141

Carrots
Buying & Storing 11
Riced 38
Juiced 39
Beef Bourguignon 108
Beef Hotpot 117
Beef Po Boys on Spinach Bun 112
Brown Butter Frosted Carrot Cake 156
Carrot Coffeecake Muffins 92
Carrot Jelly 56
Chicken Enchiladas 110
Chicken Tetrazzini with Asparagus 126
Citrus Carrot Chutney 57
Cornbread Meatloaf 112
Easy Vegetable Soup 74
Fresh Veggie Noodles 118
Grilled Vegetables 147
Homemade Chicken Pot Pie 120
Kohlrabi Chutney 58
No-Bake Carrot Peanut Butter Truffles 153
Pumpkin Beef Stew 121
Savory Mini Meat Pies 66
Shepherd's Pie 124

Shepherd's Pie Potato Skins 64
Sloppy Joes 130
Tangy Meatballs 72
Too Good to be Veggie Lasagna 113
Veggie Crust Mini Pizza 71
Veggie Peanut Chicken
   & Zucchini Noodles 122
Veggie Poppers 70

Cauliflower

Buying & Storing 12
Flour (Riced) 33
Banana Cauliflower Muffins 104
Battered Spicy Cauliflower Bites 68
Cauliflower au Gratin Pasta 137
Cauliflower Pizza Crust 82
Cauliflower Tortillas 83
Savory Cauliflower Cheeseball 65
Veggie Poppers 70
Western Beef and Corn Casserole 132

Celery

Buying & Storing 12
Minced 46
Easy Vegetable Soup 74
Chicken Enchiladas 110
Crock Pot Pasta Bolognese-style Sauce 130
Cornbread Meatloaf 112
Homemade Chicken Pot Pie 120
Savory Mini Meat Pies 66
Sloppy Joes 130

Green Peas

Buying & Storing 13
Diced 47
Beef Hotpot 117
Homemade Chicken Pot Pie 120
Kale & Pea Pesto 58
Pumpkin Beef Stew 121
Shepherd's Pie 124
Shepherd's Pie Potato Skins 64

Kale

Buying & Storing 13
Purée 48
Juice 49
Baked Beans with Kale 138
Breakfast Turnovers 96
Cheeseburger Pockets 116
Creamy Pepper Kale Mayo 60
Crockpot Breakfast Casserole 101
Fresh Veggie Noodles 118
Kale & Pea Pesto 58
Kale Coconut Cream Pie 164
Skillet Ziti with Sausage & Kale 128
Slow Cooker Tortellini Kale Soup 75
Stuffed Pasta Shells 129

Kohlrabi

Buying & Storing 14
Chopped, Roasted & Minced 36
Beef Hotpot 117
Kohlrabi and Zucchini Fritters 145
Kohlrabi Chutney 58
Kohlrabi Loaf Cake 158
Sausage & Kohlrabi Fettuccini 133

Leeks

Buying & Storing 14
Minced 34
Bacon and Cheese Quiche 100
Beef Hotpot 117
Beef Po Boys on Spinach Buns 112
Cheeseburger Pockets 116
Cornbread Meatloaf 112
Cowboy Beans 140
Crockpot Breakfast Casserole 101
Crockpot Pasta Bolognese-style Sauce 130
Easy Vegetable Soup 74
Homemade Chicken Pot Pie 120
Omelet Muffins 106
Potato Broccoli Soup 73
Pumpkin Beef Stew 121
Rutabaga Bake 142
Sausage and Chard Frittata 95
Savory Mini Meat Pies 66
Shepherd's Pie 124
Shepherd's Pie Potato Skins 64
Skillet Ziti with Sausage & Kale 128
Sloppy Joes 130
Slow Cooker Tortellini Kale Soup 75
Smooth Salsa 61
Spinach Feta Rolls 86
Veggie Crust Mini Pizza 71
Veggie Peanut Chicken
   & Zucchini Noodles 122
Western Beef and Corn Casserole 132

Onion
Buying & Storing 14
Minced 35
Bacon and Cheese Quiche 100
Beef Bourguignon 108
Beef Hotpot 117
Beef Po Boys on Spinach Buns 112
Cheeseburger Pockets 116
Cornbread Meatloaf 112
Cowboy Beans 140
Crockpot Breakfast Casserole 101
Crockpot Pasta Bolognese-style Sauce 130
Easy Vegetable Soup 74
Fiesta Corn 146
Homemade Chicken Pot Pie 120
Potato Broccoli Soup 73
Pumpkin Beef Stew 121
Sausage and Chard Frittata 95
Savory Mini Meat Pies 66
Shepherd's Pie 124
Shepherd's Pie Potato Skins 64
Skillet Ziti with Sausage & Kale 128
Sloppy Joes 130
Slow Cooker Tortellini Kale Soup 75
Smooth Salsa 61
Spinach Feta Rolls 86
Spinach Salisbury Steak 114
Veggie Crust Mini Pizza 71
Veggie Peanut Chicken
   & Zucchini Noodles 122
Western Beef and Corn Casserole 132

Pumpkin
Buying & Storing 15
Purée 40
Pumpkin Beef Stew 121
Pumpkin-Cranberry Muffins 105
Pumpkin Pull-Apart Loaf 84
Spicy Pumpkin Bread 85

Rutabaga
Buying & Storing 15
Riced & Mashed 42
Grilled Vegetables 147
Pumpkin Beef Stew 121
Rutabaga Bake 142
Shepherd's Pie 124
Sweet & Savory Squash & Root Veggies 141

Spinach
Buying & Storing 16
Purée 50
Juice 51
Bacon and Cheese Quiche 100
Bacon Spinach Pesto Roll Ups 67
Beef Po Boys on Spinach Bun 112
Cowboy Beans 140
Fresh Veggie Noodles 118
Pepperoni Spinach Roll Up 125
Spinach BBQ Baked Beans 136
Spicy Spinach Mustard 59
Spinach Buns 80
Spinach Feta Rolls 86
Spinach Salisbury Steak 114
Spinach Vanilla Cake 154
Too Good to be Veggie Lasagna 113
Veggie Crust Mini Pizza 71

Sweet Potatoes
Buying & Storing 16
Purée 41
Morning Potato Nachos 98
Sweet & Savory Squash & Root Veggies 141
Sweet Potato Cake 152
Sweet Potato Cheesecake 163
Sweet Potato Fries 148
Sweet Potato Pudding 151

Swiss Chard
Buying & Storing 17
Purée 52
Sausage and Chard Frittata 95

Tomatoes and **Cherry Tomatoes**
Buying & Storing 17
Purée 31
Roasted, Cheery 32
Chicken Enchiladas 110
Skillet Ziti with Sausage & Kale 128
Slow Cooker Tortellini Kale Soup 75
Smooth Salsa 61
Zucchini Flatbread Pizza 88

Zucchini
Buying & Storing 18
Shredded 53
Choclazini Cake 160
Easy Vegetable Soup 74
Kohlrabi and Zucchini Fritters 145
Zucchini Bread 90
Zucchini Flatbread Pizza 88
Zucchini Spice Cake 159

Cooking Measurement Equivalents

1 cup = 16 tablespoons

16 tablespoons = 48 teaspoons

¾ cup = 12 tablespoons

⅔ cup = 10 tablespoons + 2 teaspoons

½ cup = 8 tablespoons

⅓ cup = 5 tablespoons + 1 teaspoon

¼ cup = 4 tablespoons

1 pint = 2 cups

1 quart = 2 pints

1 tablespoon = 3 teaspoons

1 gallon = 16 cups

Liquid Conversions

1 cup = 8 ounces

¾ cup = 6 ounces

⅔ cup = 5⅓ ounces

½ cup = 4 ounces

¼ cup = 2 ounces

2 tablespoons = 1 ounce

Baking Conversions

9 x 13 cake pan = 12 cupcakes = 2 9" round cake pans

9" loaf pan = 12 standard muffins

12 standard muffins = 6 jumbo muffins

Emergency Substitutions

Chili Powder Oregano and cumin in equal amounts + dash of hot sauce

Cilantro Equal amount of parsley

Curry Mix ground tumeric, ginger, black pepper, coriander, cumin, and chili powder in equal amounts.

1 Egg Baking Soda and Vinegar: 1 teaspoon of baking soda mixed with 1 tablespoon of white vinegar.

1 Egg ½ mashed medium size banana.

Ginger Equal amount of cardamom

Mayonnaise 1 cup non-fat Greek yogurt *or* 1 cup sour cream = 1 cup mayonnaise

Sour Cream 1 cup non-fat Greek yogurt = 1 cup sour cream

Vegetable Oil ½ apple sauce or ½ cup beet puree = 1 cup vegetable oil

Spices
Substitutions & Alternatives

1 tablespoon of fresh herb = 1 teaspoon of dried herb

Dried herbs tend to have a stronger flavor, so less is typically needed. A general rule is that if a recipe calls for dried herbs, use three times the amount of fresh herbs.

Spice	Substitution
Allspice	Cinnamon, Cassia, Nutmeg, Mace or Cloves
Aniseed	Fennel Seed or Anise Extract
Basil	Oregano or Thyme
Cardamom	Ginger
Chili Powder	Hot Sauce plus Oregano and Cumin
Chives	Minced Green Onion, Onion, or Leek
Cilantro	Parsley
Cinnamon	Nutmeg or Allspice
Cloves	Allspice, Cinnamon or Nutmeg
Cumin	Chili Powder
Ginger	Allspice, Cinnamon, Mace or Nutmeg
Italian Seasoning	Blend of Basil, Oregano, Rosemary and Ground Red Pepper
Marjoram	Basil, Thyme or Savory
Nutmeg	Cinnamon or Ginger
Oregano	Thyme or Basil
Poultry Seasoning	Sage plus Thyme, Marjoram, Savory, Black Pepper and Rosemary
Rosemary	Thyme, Tarragon or Savory
Red Pepper	Hot Sauce or Black Pepper
Sage	Poultry Seasoning, Marjoram, or Rosemary
Thyme	Basil, Marjoram, or Oregano

About the Author

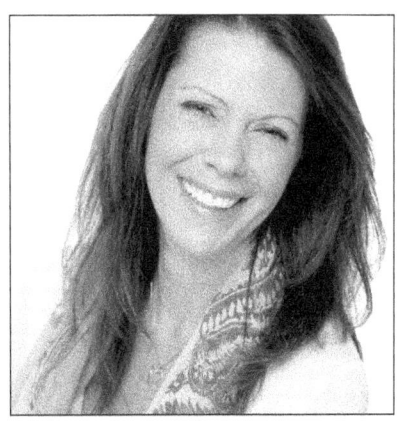

Heidi Herman is an author of books in several genres, including women's fiction, non-fiction, and children's folklore. This is her second cookbook. In 2017, she co-authored a cookbook, *Homestyle Icelandic Cooking for American Kitchens* with her mother, Íeda Jónasdóttir Herman.

Heidi was raised in Central Illinois but has made her home on a farm in South Dakota and spends winters in Arizona. In addition to writing, she loves cooking, photography, travel, and exploring the outdoors, pursuing adventure wherever she goes.

www.facebook.com/HeidihermanAuthor

www.Instagram.com/HeidihermanAuthor

website *www.HeidiHermanAuthor.com*

About the Contributor

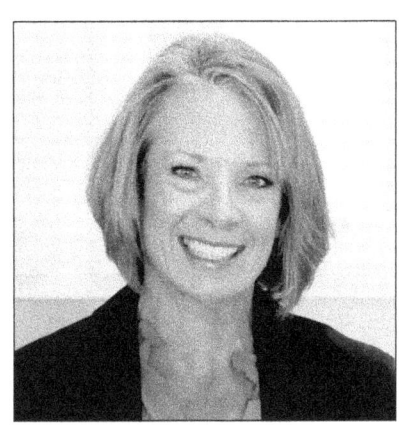

Rhonda Thornton is a National Board Certified Health and Wellness Coach, Certified Personal Trainer, and Senior Fitness Specialist with years of experience helping adults transform their health from the inside out. She specializes in habit-based coaching, strength and mobility training, and creating sustainable routines that support real life. Rhonda combines science-backed strategies with compassion and humor to help people feel better in their bodies—no matter where they're starting from. When she's not coaching or training, you'll find her entertaining, walking with her grandkids, or cheering for people taking small steps toward big change.

Other Books by Heidi Herman

Non-Fiction

On With the Butter! Spread More Living onto Everyday Life

Homestyle Icelandic Cooking for American Kitchens
(with Íeda Jónasdóttir Herman)

Women's Fiction

Her Viking Heart

Short Story Collection

The Guardians of Iceland and Other Icelandic Folk Tales

Children's Books

Yule Lads Legend: Iceland's Jólasveinar

The Icelandic Yule Lads: Mayhem at the North Pole

www.ingramcontent.com/pod-product-compliance
Lightning Source LLC
Chambersburg PA
CBHW040252090526
44586CB00043B/2930